THE PRACTITIONER'S POWER OF CHOICE
IN STAFF-DEVELOPMENT AND IN-SERVICE TRAINING

PUBLICATIONS OF THE AMSTERDAM PAEDOLOGICAL CENTER (APC)

Number 1

Series Editors:
Dr. F.X. Plooij
Prof. dr. M.G.M. van den Dungen
Drs. H.G. Helmantel
F.W. Hoogeboom

Also published by the APC in a Dutch series:
1. **Hulpverleningspraktijk en dienstverlenend onderzoek**
   Handelingsplannen en directe observaties van opvoeder-kind interactie
   F.X. Plooij en M.G.M. van der Dungen (Red.)
   1985. 198 blz. ISBN 90 265 0590 6
2. **Kwaliteit van onderwijs in het geding**
   Artikelen over onderzoek en schoolbeleid
   J.C. van der Wolf en J.J. Hox (Red.)
   1986. 160 blz. ISBN 90 265 0683 X
3. **Geïntegreerd speciaal onderwijs**
   C.M. van Rijswijk en P.J. de Kuijer (Red.)
   1987. 152 blz. ISBN 90265 0825 5
4. **Verschuivingen in orthopedagogische werkvelden**
   K. Doornbos, C.M. van Rijswijk en A.F.D. van Veen (Red.)
   1988. 202 blz. ISBN 90265 0958 8
5. **Praktijkgericht onderzoek: Debat / Design / Data**
   B.C. Swaans-Joha en J.J. Hox (Red.)
   1989. 168 blz. ISBN 90 5256 005 6

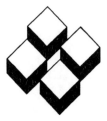

- ❖ Sociaal-agogisch Centrum,
  a residential youth care center

- ❖ E.J. van Det school for special education

- ❖ Paedological Institute
  of the City of Amsterdam

- ❖ Department of Pedagogical Sciences
  University of Amsterdam

THE PRACTITIONER'S POWER OF CHOICE
IN STAFF-DEVELOPMENT AND IN-SERVICE TRAINING

edited by:

H. K. LETICHE   Erasmus University Rotterdam / Amsterdam Polytechnic

J.C. VAN DER WOLF   University of Amsterdam

F. X. PLOOIJ   Paedological Institute of the City of Amsterdam

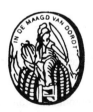

SWETS & ZEITLINGER B.V. AMSTERDAM / LISSE   PUBLISHERS

SWETS & ZEITLINGER INC. BERWYN, PA

Library of Congress Cataloging-in-Publication Data

    The Practitioner's power of choice in staff-development and in-service training /
edited by H. K. Letiche, J.C. van der Wolf, F.X. Plooij.
      p.   cm.
    Includes bibliographical references
    ISBN 90 265 1124 8
    1. Teacher--In-service training. 2. Action research in education. 3. Career
development. I. Letiche, H. K., 1946- II. Wolf, J.C. van der 1944- III. Plooij, F.X.
1946-
    LB1731.P69 1990
    371.1'46--dc20   90-10175
                                            CIP

CIP-gegevens Koninklijke Bibliotheek, Den Haag

Practitioner's

The practitioner's power of choice in staff-development and in-service training /
ed. H.K. Letiche, J.C. van der Wolf, F.X. Plooij.
– Amsterdam [etc]: Swets & Zeitlinger
– Met lit. opg.
ISBN 90-265-1124-8
SISO 450.4 UDC 37.088.6 NUGI 724
Trefw.: onderwijsresearch.

Printed in the Netherlands by Offsetdrukkerij Kanters B.V., Alblasserdam

ISBN 90 265 1124 8
NUGI 724

CONTRIBUTORS

Les Bell
Department of Education
University of Warwick
Coventry CV4 7AL
England

Christopher Day
School of Education
University of Nottingham
Nottingham NG7 2RD
England

Maarten van den Dungen
Department of Pedagogical
Sciences
University of Amsterdam
1076 CV Amsterdam
The Netherlands

Gunnar Handal
Institute for Educational
Research
University of Oslo
0317 Oslo, 3
Norway

Hugo Letiche
The Management School
Erasmus University
3000 DR Rotterdam
The Netherlands

Jennifer Nias
Cambridge Institute of
Education
Cambridge C82 2BX
England

Frans Plooij
Paedological Institute of
the City of Amsterdam
1076 CV Amsterdam
The Netherlands

Pascalle Ramaekers
Department of Pedagogical
Sciences
University of Amsterdam
1076 CV Amsterdam
The Netherlands

Fons van Wieringen
School of Education
University of Amsterdam
1015 DT Amsterdam
The Netherlands

Kees van der Wolf
Department of Pedagogical Sciences
University of Amsterdam
1076 CV Amsterdam
The Netherlands

PREFACE

This is the sixth book produced by the Foundation called the *Amsterdams Pedologisch Centrum* (APC). It is the first volume of a series to appear in English. With the year 1992 coming closer and a United Europe taking shape, the APC Foundation is broadening its horizon.

The *Amsterdams Pedologisch Centrum* Foundation is a joint venture of the following four institutes: Department of Pedagogical Sciences of the University of Amsterdam, The Paedological Institute of the City of Amsterdam (Institute of Child Studies), the E.J. van Det school for special education, and Het Sociaal-agogisch Centrum, a residential youth care center.

One of the Foundation's aims is to promote critical discussion of anything to do with the triad "innovation, research, and training" in the realms of family support, (special) education, youth care, mental retardation, and the diagnostics involved. One of the means used to further this discussion is the production of the series of books. The Foundation also organizes conferences. The production of a book is often based on or gives rise to a conference.

Although a variety of subjects have been addressed in the books making up the Dutch series, one topic emerged repeatedly: the special type of applied research that is needed to encourage and foster innovation, training, and professional development. The first volume (see list on title page) dealt mainly with direct observation of social interactions as a tool to provide feedback for planning by teachers and group leaders. The special relationship between researcher and practitioner(s) is discussed as well: ultimately, the researcher should make him- or herself superfluous; the triangular relationship between researcher, facilitator, and practitioner should become transformed into the bilateral relationship of the practitioner and the facilitator after both have familiarized themselves with the research-approach to be used. More generally, the fifth book in the series addressed the types of applied research that might be useful for practitioners.

In the present book this central topic recurs and is based firmly in the wider context of professional development and in-service training in education, and the usefulness of innovation and research is guaranteed by giving the practitioner the power of choice.

The timeliness of the concern about the quality of our education systems and the discussion in this book on finding the best ways to improve that quality, is illustrated by a few recent events. In the recent school riots in and around Paris, teachers and students alike were fighting for better working conditions. In The Netherlands the unions have been arguing in favor of the recognition of teaching as a profession as is the case for other vocations, such as law and medicine.

Since similar examples can surely be found for each and every country in Europe, it would probably pay to reach out to each other and join forces in attacking these problems. By ignoring the idiosyncracies of each country and identifying the common problems, we may learn from each other. At the moment, efforts in Europe are scattered. In various if not all of the countries people are facing the same problems and inventing the same wheel time and time again.

Apart from the lack of communication between countries, there are gaps between the various professions dealing with education. This problem is addressed at great length in this book. Admittedly, in a wide variety of learned, international societies researchers meet and exchange results. But it is rare for practitioners, trainers, and researchers to meet for a common purpose. Scientists and practitioners live in different worlds and often are not very familiar with how the others are tackling the same problem they themselves are dealing with. To eliminate this lack of communication between countries and professions, the I.E.D.P.E. (*Institut Européen pour le développement des potentialités de tous les enfants* = European Institute for development of the potential of all children) was founded a little more than one year ago in Paris. The IEDPE sees a solution in the use of the network approach. The Institute has united scientists and practitioners from all European countries to deal with the major threats to the development of all children.

Let us hope that this book will make at least a small contribution to this new European movement.

January 1991

Frans X. Plooij
Maarten G.M. van den Dungen
Harm G. Helmantel
Frank W. Hoogeboom

CONTENTS

Contributors

Preface

Introduction   11

Part I Description of practitioner research

1. How practitioners are silenced, how practitioners
    are empowered   19
    Jennifer Nias

2. Only connect... relationships between higher
    education and schools   37
    Christopher Day

3. Promoting the articulation of tacit knowledge
    through the counselling of practitioners   71
    Gunnar Handal

**Part II Various approaches to the professional development of
teachers and schools**

4. The provision of professional development for
    teachers   87
    Les Bell

5. Transferring practitioner research   117
    Hugo Letiche

**Part III In-service training and staff-development in
the Netherlands**

6. Eductional policy for school development   141
    Fons van Wieringen

7. Social scientists as sorcerer's apprentices:
    The polluted relations between practitioners and experts   149
    Maarten van den Dungen

8. The development of professional competence and interaction:
    New goals for in-service traning and staff-development   163
    Kees van der Wolf & Pascalle Ramaekers

Bibliography   177

INTRODUCTION

Hugo Letiche, Erasmus University Rotterdam, Amsterdam
  Polytechnic
Kees van der Wolf, University of Amsterdam
Frans Plooij, Paedological Institute of the City of Amsterdam

Practitioners in education work in a glass house. Almost everyone in a Western industrialized country has spent an appreciable proportion of his youth in school. Thus, many of them feel themselves to some degree qualified to participate in discussions on the quality of education and of those employed in the field of education. Certainly, those who are confronted with school affairs via their children have a tendency to hold very strong opinions. Parents always want the best for their children. They realize that achievement in school strongly determines the prospects of those children. Should the child fail to do well, we blame not ourselves but the school.

In most of the countries of Europe, much is said, and complained, about the level of the teachers. Teaching is said to have been better in the past. This must partially be ascribed to nostalgic thinking, in which youthful experiences are idealized. It is sometimes forgotten that in both Europe and the United States of America, a much higher percentage of the children go on to higher education than was formerly the case. From American data it is known that in 1940 only 25% of the adults had a high-school diploma; in 1980, this percentage had risen to 68.7; and in 1982 to 71. A similar trend can be seen in Europe as well. This is not the place to discuss the political and cultural factors responsible for the demand for better education, although it may be said that the quality of schooling has improved and that this quality is more evenly distributed over the population.

Rightly or wrongly, the quality of education and of educators is often judged negatively. With respect to the improvement of quality desired by many, a discussion has arisen about the assignment of funds for supplementary and further education in the educational system. It is argued that such funds should go directly to the schools or the appropriate authorities. This is seen as the best way to solve the problem. It is assumed that schools and their boards know best what would be good for them, and if they as clients have free access to funds, qualitatively excellent supplementary and further education will emerge soon enough, according to the time-honoured market mechanism of supply and demand. It is of course a sobering thought that in the decentralization of the management of supplementary and further education a role is played, and possibly a leading role, by efforts to reduce the costs of innovative education.

New chances are at hand! And danger as well. For there is a risk that in the haste to capture part of the market as supplier, precedence will be given to the development of traditional curricula of the kind that gave rise to dissatisfaction in the past. And even if qualitatively poor curricula disappear in the long run as a result of the market mechanism, it may still be asked whether the field must in the short run be burdened by supplementary educational products that have proved unusable.

One obstacle encountered in setting up adequate courses in the field of further education is the frequently observed ambivalent attitude of practitioners with respect to the knowledge and skills of educators trained in the social sciences. On the one hand, there is a certain respect for the results of the "official sciences", and on the other hand, there is often indifference for the theories that seem to be so widely separated from practice. In The Netherlands and elsewhere, this process of mutual alienation has often been described. The scientist does not asign sufficient importance to the voice of the practitioner, with the result that the latter has less and less to say (the expert as "silencer" and the practitioner as "silenced").

Much of this situation can be traced to the historical developments in fields of those disciplines, which were long devoted to the formulation of grand theories. The arrival of the empirical-analytical movement in the field of education and pedagogy gave rise to immense optimism about the possibility of solving every kind of educational and pedagogical problem by scientific methods. This optimism often proved unwaranted: it delivered education into the hands of technocrats and "measurement maniacs" with little feeling for what the true essence of education is all about. These researchers had little practical knowledge. The reaction to all this gave rise to a movement back to the teacher in the classroom. How could he or she be involved in the development of insights leading to better working methods in education? How could teachers be encouraged to define a general policy? How could the growth of individual teachers be promoted without hindrance to this "school-based" curriculum-development"? In short, how can innovation, research, and training attain a better balanced co-existence?

On April 6, 1990, a congress initiated by the *Amsterdams Pedologisch Centrum* was held in Amsterdam. Invited speakers were asked to deal with the following themes:

1. How can the gap between science and practice in the fields of supplementary and further education be filled?

2. What has been done in this area in The Netherlands and elsewhere, and to what extent can that be adapted for The Netherlands?
3. In connection with Europe after 1992, how are educational problems comparable with those of The Netherlands being handled?

This volume contains the papers presented by a number of the invited experts to the congress.

What elements, it might be asked, will be crucial in producing or hindering rapport between text and reader? That the ideas are practical? That the writing be clear and accessible? That the authors' voices are felt present and evoke a sympathetic response? That the text reads easily? That the audience is already dealing with the issues under discussion?

One can be certain that:

— the theme of how to organize the further education and training of in-service professionals is actual;
— the decision to Europeanize the discussion reflects what is to come;
— the authors do not hide behind academic personas, but are up-front about their ideas;
— the programs described have been successfully applied, the proposals made are realizable.

But it is known that resistance to the commitment of the authors to the principle of the *reflective practitioner* exists. Much training is instrumental and utilitarian in character; it offers skill-training via continuing vocational education. Trainees practice professional competences which have been identified as crucial to success. The quick-fix, tell-them-what-they-should-do, brand of training has many adherents. Performativity – the quickest way of doing something with the least energy – is often the goal of in-service programmes. This book is rooted in a tradition which embraces the classical pedagogical values of *human speculation, experiential, insight* and *personal motivation*. Its social and educational ethics are irrelevant for the dissemination and distribution strategy of (most of) the training industry. The mercantilization of training is ill-served by this book. Practitioner research is strong in dialogue involvement and innovation; weak in rules, guidelines, and routines. In this book the writers describe bricolage:with a few recognizable basic tools, drawn from qualitative and exploratory research, they undertake concrete practical projects with practitioners. It is hoped that the respect for context and the personal dynamics of professional cooperation has made it possible for each project described here to be unique and exciting. When we first began to bundle our forces to hold a working conference and to prepare this book, our project had the nick-name: "Silencers and the silenced". Practitioners – teachers in their classrooms, school faculties in their staff rooms, educational authorities in their offices – have been *silenced*. Their voices are absent from the professional pedagogic literature. The group which seemingly has jammed the practitioner's voice is that of the academic pedagogues. The *silencers* do research and give expert advice; the practitioners experience that research and advice (mostly) as alien to themselves. Although the theme of silencers and the silenced has persisted throughout the project, we decided that it would be excessively negative to permit it to predominate. After all, there are responses and answers to the theory/practice dilemma, as well as collaboration and dialogue between practitioners and pedagogues. Thus, the book is the product of a shared concern for the quality of the practitioner/pedagogue relationship and has itself emerged as a statement in affirmation of practitioner/pedagogue cooperation.

It is one of the authors' goals that via this book practitioner research will become a social realm that is more recognizable and knowable for the reader. The further professionalization of teachers as described here offers pedagogues the chance to develop their interactive integrity and practitioners a way to bring in-service activity closer to their chosen goals.

The book is divided into three parts. In the first part, practitioner research is described in all its facets. In the first chapter, Jennifer Nias describes her commitment to practitioner research: that commitment is grounded in her fundamental respect for teachers and their sensibility. She acknowledges the general tension between academic pedagogues and practicing teachers and uses that to describe the efforts to overcome it. Her creative resolution for what she sees as an unnecessary conflict becomes clear. The energy and enthusiasm of the British teacher-as-researcher movement is admirably portrayed in Nias' text.

Chris Day, in the second chapter, reviews his long experience with practitioner research and summarizes for us what he found to be three crucial exemplary illustrations of teacher research. His examples highlight the similarities and differences between individual and group projects. Various facets of the rewards of practitioner research are described: individual personal, professional in-service, organizational school-wide, and faculty team development are illustrated.

Gunnar Handal concludes the initial trio of descriptive chapters. He draws on his experience as a facilitator of teacher professional development. He describes how in Norway he investigates in-service reality cooperatively with teachers. He points out which questions about practice are easily answered and which are stumbling blocks. He demonstrates how collaborative research stretches teacher professionalism to entertain and answer questions which would otherwise not be addressed at all.

In Part Two, Les Bell kicks off the first of two chapters that remain fairly descriptive, but focus on the broader categorization of practitioner research. Bell asks himself what sorts of practitioner professionalization have emerged from the teacher-directed approach in the last twenty-five years. What have been the strengths and weaknesses, the factors emphasized or neglected in the various approaches? He has given a stimulating overview of pedagogic practice that clarifies the changes in training which have taken place.

In the fifth chapter, Hugo Letiche presents a conceptual model of practitioner research which he believes clarifies this field of practice without unduly simplifying it. He defines and explores the demands made on teachers and pedagogues before practitioner research can be effective. He deals with ideas or assumptions that have given support to practitioner research and asks himself whether these prerequisites remain relevant today. Finally, he addresses the question of transferring practice, as described in the book, to The Netherlands.

In Part Three, the sixth, seventh, and eighth chapters address changes, challenges, and issues in the professionalization of teachers in The Netherlands.

Fons van Wieringen describes Dutch policy on teacher professionalization, focussing on the implied, human resource management issues. He describes the traditional policy weaknesses and indicates which issues are currently actual.

Maarten van den Dungen discusses the divorce of pedagogics (rooted in research and empirical investigation) and practice (based on in-service experience). He criticizes the unsatisfactory effort to allow theory to lead practice in technology, and proposes a cooperative training model combining on-the-job learning with theoretical rigor.

Kees van der Wolf and Pascalle Ramaekers have attempted a synthesis between practitioner research and Dutch practice. They indicate how the ideas presented could contribute to the professionalization of Dutch teachers and search for a form of institutionalization which would maximize the chances of success.

Without the support and encouragement of the *Amsterdams Pedologisch Centrum* Foundation, the department of Pedagogical Sciences of the *University of Amsterdam*, the *Amsterdam Polytechnic* and the *Erasmus University Rotterdam* this project would never have reached fruition. The two teaching assistents, René van Hattem and Peter Walop, guided the conference through many organizational snares, earning our gratitude.

❖ I ❖

DESCRIPTION OF PRACTITIONER RESEARCH

HOW PRACTITIONERS ARE SILENCED, HOW PRACTITIONERS ARE EMPOWERED

Jennifer Nias, Cambridge Institute of Education

This chapter is structured around two main questions: Do academics prevent practitioners from speaking confidently about their own experience and if so, how? Is it possible for academics to help practitioners find and express a professional voice? An attempt to answer these questions leads into a discussion of a possible future partnership between the two. Before that, however, I make four introductory points.

First, the conference from which this chapter grew was concerned with the relationship between teachers and pedagogues (I use the term interchangeably with 'academics' and 'educational researchers'). However, coming from the United Kingdom, I feel it important to say that there are others who have as great a potential to stifle the voice of the practitioners as have academics. English politicians have gone a long way in the past decade towards taking both power and influence away from teachers. The latter have no bargaining rights in relation to their pay or salary structure and have had conditions of service imposed upon them. State schools now have a national curriculum and national assessment. The structure and content of both have been established with minimal consultation. Most educational policy decisions are made and administered centrally; the Education Act of 1988 gave the Secretary of State for Education individual powers which exceed those of all other ministers except the Prime Minister. Furthermore, as part of this legislation the governing bodies of individual schools have been given extensive powers and responsibilities over the funding and staffing of those schools, yet teachers have only a minimal representation on such bodies. Moreover, while teacher autonomy is reduced and undermined in these and other ways, they are publicly attacked by politicians and by much of the media, and are held responsible by both for many of the country's social and economic problems. Not surprisingly, many teachers feel that it is for political rather than educational reasons that they are increasingly being denied a voice in both policy and practice.

The second point I wish to make may seem to contradict this. Anyone with a personal knowledge of teachers, knows that in one important sense they have never been silenced. As the title of my recent book (Primary Teachers Talking, Nias, 1989) suggests, when teachers meet one another or anyone who is interested in listening to them, they talk about their work – fluently, intelligently, relentlessly. There is no shortage of discussion among teachers. Indeed, one effect of the introduction of a national curriculum into English schools has been to increase the staff's need and desire to talk to one another, about pupils' learning, about curriculum, about pedagogy. Our concern should not be to start teachers talking, since such an aspiration would be redundant, but to ensure that someone other than their co-professionals is listening.

Thirdly, I need to point out that, as far as I know, no research exists which substantiates the claims that I and many other English pedagogues would wish to make on behalf of teacher research (though see Dadds, in progress, and Ovens, in progress). I can speak from the experience of myself and my colleagues, but the whole subject lacks detailed and objective evaluation. Such an enquiry would serve teacher educators and teachers well, giving them information through which practice could be improved and still more effective partnerships be built. Without it, arguments about teacher research cannot move far beyond the realms of hypothesis, conjecture, assertion and belief.

My last introductory remarks concern myself, since my readers' capacity to hear what I wish to say may be affected by the sort of person they deem me to be. Three sets of facts may be relevant. First, I have an impeccable academic background; a first degree (in history) from the University of Oxford, a doctorate (in the sociology of education, acquired nearly twenty years later) from the University of California at Berkeley, and a lengthy list of publications. The second is that I trained as a primary school teacher after taking my first degree and chose to return to primary teaching after completing my doctorate. I have been committed for most of my working life to improving and facilitating the education of young children and have had the opportunity to become steeped in both the practice and theory of education. My third point arises from this: I have never been convinced that the distinction which both pedagogues and teachers draw between these two aspects of our shared avocation are valid ones. As a school teacher, I always thought, often in quite abstract terms, about what I was doing and looked for generalizable patterns in it. As an academic and a teacher educator, my concern was, for many years, to use and sometimes to generate theory which might be helpful to teachers, and, more recently, to assist them in making their own. My desire to help teachers acquire a professional voice to which others will listen stems, I suspect, from a lifelong desire to effect a public reconciliation between parts of myself which I feel to be in harmony but which educationalists commonly set in opposition to one another.

Practitioners silenced

To turn to my first main question: Do academics prevent practitioners from speaking confidently about their own experience and if so, how?

My answer would be that, in general, they do, but that many teachers collude in their own enforced silence. Academic domination of educational research is seldom challenged by classroom practitioners who may indeed find it a convenient defence for their professional conservatism.

Traditionally, academics, like the educational research and theory which they produce, are perceived by practitioners as remote and as threatening. Remoteness has many causes. Pedagogues and educational researchers belong to organizations and institutions with distinctive histories, sometimes they have separate occupational trainings and even when pedagogues are drawn from schools, they have to accept a different culture when they change their jobs. Most teachers meet academics only as the tutors of their initial or in-service courses, as the authors of the books which they are recommended to read on these courses or as 'experts' visiting their schools in order to undertake research in them. As a result, pedagogues are often perceived as personally remote from teachers and certainly as far removed from the 'chalk face' of the classroom. Furthermore, as theoreticians, and particularly as researchers, they use methods and, above all, a language which many teachers experience as esoteric and, all too often, as incomprehensible. I remember the concern I felt when, five years ago, I had written an introductory booklet for the schools in which I and two colleagues were to work on a research project. I then asked a teacher friend to check it for me. She gave it back to me saying, "I don't understand parts of this. I'm afraid you speak a different language to me." Yet I had laboured to make it 'user-friendly'! This problem is exaggerated when researchers write in an academic register for fellow pedagogues. I and my colleagues find a continuing difficulty in persuading teachers on in-service courses to read educational books or papers, not because the content is irrelevant to their concerns but because of the ways in which this literature is structured and written. The distance between the daily worlds, the occupational concerns, the interests and the professional language of academics and teachers would not by itself deprive teachers of a voice. Unfortunately, status is also differentially distributed, almost always in favour of academics. The latter's interest in pupils' learning, in teachers' actions, in the work of schools can easily be construed as attempts to de-skill teachers: to take away from them their monopoly of expert knowledge of, for example, individual children and how they learn, of the choice of curriculum content and how best to teach it, of school organization and its impact on different pupils.

This potential threat shows itself in three main ways. Because academics claim, or are seen to claim, to have access to information about children, curriculum, teaching methods, school organization which is more detailed, accurate and insightful than that of teachers, they seem to deny the validity of practitioners' knowledge, and so to undermine their status as experts in the job which they do. By the same token, researchers implicitly deny teachers' ability to generate knowledge, since by definition knowledge is that which academics produce. Thirdly, since researchers have a vested interest in generalising, they underplay the significance and complexity of individual cases: children become 'types', behaviours are placed in categories. As a result, teachers' daily experience of particular children and of the way in which they adapt and select in order to facilitate their pupils' learning is undervalued.

To deny teachers' ability to 'know' and to create 'knowledge' is also to threaten their status, self-esteem and self-confidence. The status which accrues in our society from access to knowledge is a source of influence and, often, of power. So, academics have the capacity to tell teachers that they are behaving in ways which are ineffectual, inefficient or even morally wrong, and to do this in a language which teachers themselves have difficulty in understanding. Examples in my professional lifetime are the rival polemics which have arisen from academic debates over 'child-centredness', 'cultural deprivation', the epistemology of the curriculum, psycholinguistic approaches to the teaching of reading, behaviour modification. Readers will be able to supply other examples from their own experience.

Sometimes too academics go beyond an implicit attack on existing practice and redefine what it is that teachers should be doing. Their own conviction about a particular topic may be so deep that it assumes the nature of a mission. Under these circumstances they often appear to practitioners to be holding up a model of ideal attitudes, thinking or behaviour, without giving any indication of how this might be achievcd ("following children's interests", "teaching for understanding", would be examples). Yet academic crusades which are supported by the heavy investment of political and economic resources can be even more threatening than those which set out abstract goals. Faced with the energetic activity of committed advisers or inspectors, with well-resourced in-service training, with differentiated salary awards, with curriculum resources or packages, teachers may find it quite difficult to resist theoretically-derived models or, if they do, to avoid feeling defensive or guilty about their resistance.

Lastly, power differentials are often emphasised in western society in mundane but important ways. Pedagogues and teachers have separate salary structures and conditions of service, are often addressed by distinctive titles, tend to dress differently, to work in buildings with different characteristics. Almost always, these occupational distinctions favour academics rather than teachers (though recent pay awards in England have discriminated against pedagogues and in favour of school 'managers', such as headteachers).

However, it does not follow that all teachers are opposed to the relative power and status of academics. Much has been written about the traditional culture of teachers, especially in elementary (North America) and primary (UK) schools (eg. Waller, 1961; Jackson, 1968; Lortie, 1975; King, 1978; Woods, 1979; Hargreaves, 1980; Pollard, 1985; Simons, 1985; Nias, 1987b, 1989; Lieberman, 1988). Different in emphasis though each of these studies is, together they paint a picture of teaching as a conservative occupation whose traditional culture favours individualism, privacy and practical knowledge, which sets a high priority upon hierarchy and a sense of feeling in control and in which work is characterised by immediacy, complexity and affective rather than material or intellectual rewards. It is not surprising that it should also therefore be an oral rather than a written culture, and one which is characterised by a professional epistemology which stresses the individual case rather than shared technical understanding.

Educational research and theory which purport to address universals, and from which general prescriptions can be derived, threaten this traditional culture in several ways. They challenge the primacy of the individual and of his/her craft knowledge, they reduce the perceived complexity of the task, they elevate the intellectual above both the practical and the affective; and, especially when undertaken by people who are perceived as more powerful than teachers, they threaten the latter's sense of control. It may therefore be the case that teachers find it convenient to dismiss the work of academics as irrelevant, incomprehensible and remote from reality. Perhaps the gap which exists between pedagogues and teachers cannot be bridged by the former acting on their own. We must hold open the possibility that teachers reject the potential value of educational theory, and do not heed the findings of educational research, because these assail their traditional culture. It may be that there is more than one reason why teachers talk to each other rather than in a more public forum. To be sure they are often silenced by academics, but it is also possible that by colluding in this silence, they can preserve a sense of expertise, of autonomy, and even of power.

Teacher research

Faced with these formidable obstacles, is it possible for pedagogues to help practitioners find and express a professional voice? However, before I directly address my second main question I would like to suggest that we should not throw the baby out with the bath water, especially where in-service teacher education is concerned. Over the years, individual teachers have been empowered and given a voice by induction into academic modes of thinking and expression. To be sure, this process resembles certain forms of colonialism in which the 'assimilés' are given the status and privileges of the imperial power. There are those who reject it for this reason, arguing that it preserves and strengthens the hegemony of a particular group and of the values which they espouse. I take a different view, suggesting that until teachers can and are willing to speak for themselves in a manner which will be heeded by theoreticians and decision-makers outside schools, it would be foolish to block a channel of communication which has served, and continues to serve, to give a minority of teachers a voice in another culture and to ensure that the views of practitioners are represented, albeit through a means and in a language to which all of them do not have access. Teachers will not find their own voice by rejecting the one which academics offer them, but rather by absorbing it and adapting it to their own circumstances and their own ends.

For the rest of this chapter, I focus upon a possible redefinition of the relationship between academics and teachers, arguing that despite the criticisms which can justly be made of it, teacher research offers a way forward, towards a partnership between theoreticians and practitioners. First, I offer a definition and a brief history of teacher research, then I outline the criticisms which have been made of it, before examining its strengths and commenting upon possible future developments. By teacher research I understand: deliberate, systematic and rigorous enquiry by practitioners into their own practices, understandings and situations. Its aim is the improvement of these practices, understandings and situations, so that pupils' education may be enhanced and the overall quality of schools' educational provision can be improved. Some (eg Carr & Kemmis, 1986) argue that practitioner research is most empowering when it is undertaken with other school members, because the collaborative process:

– stimulates debate about ends as well as means,
– offers mutual challenge to taken-for-granted assumptions and perspectives, and
– provides support for action.

While many of these claims contain a good deal of truth (Nias, 1987a & b) I suggest that teacher research can also usefully be undertaken by individuals and sometimes in cooperation with 'outsiders'.

Defined in this way, there is an obvious overlap between teacher research and action research. I prefer to use the former term for three main reasons. First, teacher enquiries do not always lead to action, certainly not to immediate action. Rather, they may enhance understanding or change attitudes, both of which may mature only slowly and tentatively into changes in behaviour. Similarly, teacher enquiry cannot and should not always conform to the classic action research cycle: plan, act, observe, reflect, revised plan. It is often a messier, more complex process than this. Thirdly, there is no consensus about the meaning of 'action research', and in particular about its implicit political affiliations. I do not propose to go into this topic here, but a very clear explanation and summary of the three main types of action research is to be found in Oja and Smulyan (1989). The picture is complicated by the emergence of action research in Austria (eg. Altrichter & Posch, 1989, Kroath, 1989) Australia (Carr & Kemmis, 1986), Canada (Carson and Couture, 1988), England (Stenhouse, 1971, 1975; Elliott, 1976, 1987); and its merging in the USA with the 'reflective practitioner' movement (Schon, 1983, 1987). In each country it has acquired its own proponents, histories and shades of meaning. The time has passed when one could speak of 'action research' and be understood in the same way by all one's listeners. I therefore prefer not to use the term.

My own experience of teacher research is mainly in the context of award-bearing courses (Nias & Groundwater Smith, 1988). However, teacher research in the UK goes back at least to Lawrence Stenhouse's Humanities Curriculum Project (1967-72) at the University of East Anglia; it has been supported by the Classroom Action Research Project (CARN), initiated by John Elliott and housed since 1976 at the Centre for Applied Research in Education, University of East Anglia and the Cambridge Institute of Education. In the past 15 years it has been widely used on courses at the Cambridge Institute of Education and at many other institutions of higher education. It has found its way through such activities into many forms of school development and in-service education. All over the UK, in varied contexts, teachers are addressing their own problems and seeking to improve their own practice through the use of enquiries which they have designed and carried out themselves. Unfortunately, though I make this assertion, I cannot demonstrate its truth. As far as I know, no attempt has yet been made to plot the incidence of teacher research in the UK or to establish the uses to which it has been put. Yet I can say from recent personal experience that ex-graduates of courses from the Centre for Applied Research in Education and the Cambridge Institute of Education often base post-experience training for their colleagues on the research principles which they themselves experienced as students on our courses. It does appear that teacher research offers practitioners an educational experience which they then seek to use and foster in their work with others.

In that process we, as academics, may be asked to act as formal or informal consultants, or to make the occasional input. In general, however, our main role is as teachers of post-experience courses lasting from 40 hours to 240 hours, for part-time students working sometimes on day release but predominantly in their own time (eg. evenings, Saturdays). My chief involvement in teacher research is still as a pedagogue, as one who plans, teaches and assesses courses which help teachers in all kinds of institution to enquire into issues which they have defined themselves and to find ways of acting upon these. These courses have high academic standards as well as a practical emphasis.

Teacher research has been subjected to four main types of criticism. In summary:

There is little published evidence that teacher research is any more effective in changing practice than more accepted methods of professional development have been. It perpetuates the traditional craft culture of teaching by encouraging innovative staff members to isolate themselves in a hegemonic alliance with like-minded academics. It encourages professional myopia. It is difficult to do, and especially to do well.

There are scattered accounts by teachers of specific pieces of action research (eg Nixon, 1980; Hustler, Cassidy and Cuff, 1984; Woods, 1989). These demonstrate how the processes of hypothesis-formation, data collection and analysis have affected the thinking of individuals and encouraged them to change their practice. However, in the absence of any systematic evaluation of the effect of teacher research upon professional behaviour or upon the quality of pupils' learning experiences, such evidence as does exist is to be found only in such accounts.

It is also sometimes alleged that teacher researchers, having learnt new skills and a new language of discourse in institutions of higher education, then fail to use these to effect change in their own schools. Instead they enter into a tacit alliance with 'emancipatory' academics who become parasitic upon their efforts to undertake school-based research or to theorise about it. New courses are developed in higher education, teacher educators build fresh reputations upon their innovative practice and begin to make it public (Nias & Groundwater Smith, 1988, is a good example of this process), students become coopted and expend their energies on discussions about, for example, methodologies, power structures which inhibit change in schools, academic or political hegemonies and the need to subvert or overthrow them. Together, pedagogues and academics develop a new language, fresh theoretical concerns, different criteria for success. Conversation within such groups is often very challenging, membership of them is stimulating, ideas are bold and iconoclastic. It is easy for participants to feel that they are breaking new educational ground and to overlook the fact that they are so preoccupied with developing fresh theories that they have omitted to take any action. At its worst, two or more leading teachers in a school may form a new elite, bound together by perspectives and a discourse which they share with their academic colleagues but which alienates them from the rest of their staff. Now, a culture built upon the values of teacher research, with its emphasis upon the examination of practice, its challenge to the taken-for-granted, the high priority that it places upon change and often collaboration, is as alien to the craft culture of teachers as is the traditional academic culture. It is in the majority's interests, therefore, to marginalise their innovative colleagues, implicitly encouraging them to restrict the practice of their new skills and understandings to their own narrow circle. I have seen this happen; the existence of teachers who are committed to the improvement of practice through school-based research does not necessarily lead to widespread change in a school. Indeed, it does not even guarantee limited improvements, if the teacher-researchers confuse discussion of theoretical issues with action and never get beyond debating questions of, for example, issue-selection, validity or methodology.

A third criticism made of teacher research is that it makes the profession more susceptible to external control, in particular by encouraging practitioners to look inwards, towards the micro, while distracting their attention from the macro, and especially from structural constraints which bear upon them. Doubts of this kind offer a caricature of the teacher who, with a large class, scarce resources, in a crumbling school building with a head who is preoccupied with fund-raising and staff shortages, occupies herself with counting how many open or closed questions she uses.

Similarly, this kind of professional myopia is held to distract practitioners from considering ends, diverting them instead into a technical consideration of means. By encouraging them to focus upon their own practice it also sustains the private, individualistic, territorial values underlying the traditional culture of teaching and reduces the likelihood of strong joint action. Together these criticisms call in question the ability of teacher researchers to address fundamental problems facing schools and therefore to effect radical change in them. A related concern is potential teacher vulnerability: self-study and self-portrayal, it is claimed, open teachers' practice up to the gaze of hostile critics who can use the information generated by teacher-researchers to appraise, sanction and control, rather than to offer help and guidance. Viewed this way, teacher research can be seen as the pedagogical equivalent of politically motivated self-accusation and confession. So, teacher research can be attacked on two conflicting sets of grounds – that it makes professional behaviour both too finely-focussed and private, and too public. In either case, teachers themselves are blinded to the constraints which operate upon them.

The last main critique of the notion of teacher as researcher is different in kind from the others. Whereas the first three focus upon the apparent ineffectuality of structured self-study in bringing about change in schools, the last emphasises the specialised nature of research and the difficulties which teachers encounter in doing it well. Various arguments are advanced. Some of them come from pedagogues. For example: teaching and research are both demanding occupations and no one can do simultaneous justice to them; teachers find it hard to read and write in an academic register; practitioners cannot overcome the problems of validity and reliability which are inherent in self-study; 'outsiders' can see more clearly than 'insiders' what aspects of a social situation most call for enquiry; 'insiders' cannot be frank about their findings because they must continue to live and work with their colleagues.

Moreover, teachers themselves are often anxious about their perceived inadequacy as researchers and particularly about their likely inability to meet traditional academic standards. Where research is conceived, in Stenhouse's terms (Rudduck and Hopkins, 1985) as "systematic enquiry made public", the last stage of this process presents particular difficulties. The traditional isolation, self-referent-ialism and authority dependence of the profession lead many practitioners to feel that they have nothing of significance to say to anyone else about their practice. Furthermore, their tendency to define their pupils and the learning context as unique and complex, makes them reluctant to accept that their experience may be generalisable. They therefore distrust the value of making public their studies of individual cases. This argument is sometimes also used as a circular one, defend-ing and enhancing the privacy of the teaching act: each teacher's behaviour and situation is unique and generalizations about teaching and learning are therefore impossible. Because generalizations cannot be made, there is no need to make public the insights individuals derive from self-study. Therefore, systematic enquiry does not need to be made public.

In my experience, teachers are often reluctant to write, more especially in an orthodox academic format and style. Their reluctance raises other questions: What public outcomes should research have? For example, must these always be written or is there scope for audio-tape, video tape and photography? Who should be the prime audience for research reports (eg. colleagues, administrators or academics)? What effect should the answer to this question have upon the length, form and style of written submissions? What is the place and function of narrative, should it be accompanied by analysis and if so, how best can these approaches be combined? Lack of resolution of these and similar problems lends weight to the accusation that teachers can seldom become 'good' insider-researchers. It also impedes progress towards new forms of 'systematic enquiry made public'. In the meantime, the time-consuming and difficult nature of 'academic' writing gives teachers and academics a sound excuse to collude in maintaining the hegemony which has traditionally controlled the nature and direction of educational research and theory.

It will be obvious by now that I do not see teacher research as a proven panacea or as a simple recipe for school improvement. Nor do I regard academic involvement in, or sponsorship of it as an unmixed blessing. Having made these two points clear, I now return to the notion of partnership, to my second main question: Is it possible for academics to help practitioners find and express a professional voice?

Practitioners empowered

Despite the lack of published evidence, and subject to the doubts I have expressed above, my answer to the second main question is, yes, it is. I shall first lay out my reasons for saying this and, second, comment upon the potential for development which exists in the relationship between these two groups of educationalists. In his Chapter (in this volume), Les Bell examines some of the ways in which cooperation between academics and at least a minority of practitioners may be, and in practice sometimes is, accomplished. Accordingly, I have not addressed this topic here.

In my experience, school-based research strengthens the teachers' voice in three main ways. The first – self-confidence – underpins and goes hand in hand with the other two. Often for the first time in their professional lives, practitioners are asked to decide for themselves what are the issues which they feel to be important, to pinpoint the aspects of their practice and their professional contexts about which they require further information. The issues they choose may at first sight seem to an outsider to be relatively trivial – Why can I seldom work undisturbed with one group of pupils? Why do our staff meetings never finish on time? What use is made by which pupils of the different resource areas in the classroom? – but they represent for the practitioner an important shift from an external to an internal locus of control. Similarly, the fact that teachers often find a productive answer to the questions they have set themselves gives them an increased sense of efficacy. The process of rigorously gathering, examining and analysing evidence about themselves, their behaviours and their contexts also helps them to be able to speak with conviction about what they believe and what they do. Furthermore, they learn, or are reminded, that they can be self-determining learners, that they can acquire knowledge, insights, understandings, and sometimes skills through their own efforts and enquiries. Equally important, they learn that they can withstand and overcome the profound sense of disequilibrium which frequently arises from systematically examining one's own practice and from having to question the basic assumptions on which one's professional behaviour is built.

Now, second only to fatigue, teachers' greatest enemies are their chronic guilt and self-doubt (I have examined the reasons for and manifestations of this feeling in Nias, 1989). A more or less permanent sense of inadequacy, coupled with a respect for authority, leaves them vulnerable to persuasion and control by outside agencies. I have already suggested that academics and, more recently, politicians are the main groups who affect teachers in this way. In my experience teachers who have engaged in school-based research, especially when this is collaborative, are more ready to question the expectations and demands which others place upon them, than those who have never been given the opportunity to examine and reflect upon their own practice. A recent example springs to mind: the Education Act 1988, requires schools to produce development plans, and many local authorities, assisted by academics, have offered headteachers and teachers a model to use in undertaking this institutional review. A headteacher on a Cambridge Institute of Education Advanced Diploma course chose to study the process by which her school development plan was being made and implemented. She found, to her initial consternation, that it bore little resemblance to the tidy cyclical model of needs identification, action planning, action and review which had been pressed upon her from above by a combination of academics and local authority officers. Having documented the beneficial effects upon her staff of their own messy, complex, pragmatic adaptation of the official model, she is now prepared to question the latter and to point up its theoretical and practical limitations.

As teachers become more aware of what they are thinking, planning and doing, and are able to substantiate their claims to knowledge with evidence that they have helped to gather, they become more able to talk about it to others. Knowing what one wants to say is a necessary condition for saying it clearly. My claim is that teacher research improves the individual's capacity to communicate, in spoken and in written words; self-confidence encourages articulacy.

The second main benefit which teachers appear to derive from being researchers is an enhanced awareness of the complexity of the job that they do, and the contexts in which they do it. It is a frequent, rueful comment by students on our courses that they do not learn answers but only how to ask questions; or, put another way, that every time they solve a problem, they uncover a dozen more. Learning to see problems from many angles, and so to live with ambiguity and uncertainty are important accomplishments for teachers, conditioned as they are by their traditional culture to seek control. This capacity is particularly valuable in Britain at a time of rapid social, political, environmental, as well as educational, change.

Related to these developments is an increased consciousness that interdependence and complexity are closely related, that the elements of any situation may fit together in many ways and affect one another in still more. This awareness frequently leads teachers to reflect upon their own professional contexts and in particular upon their interdependence with their colleagues. I would not argue, as Carr and Kemmis (1986) do, that teacher research must necessarily be collaborative. However, I accept that it often becomes so and that it is most effective when it involves others, or at least is undertaken with their support. There are two main reasons for this. The first is socio-psychological: without the challenge offered by other people's perspectives, it is often very difficult to uncover one's own assumptions, blindspots and biases (Nias, 1987b, summarised in Nias, 1987a, examines the crucial part which a group of peers may play in helping individual teachers to 'see anew'). The second is structural: individuals who start by enquiring into a situation in their own classrooms often discover that they cannot take the action which the logic of their research dictates because of school resources or policies or the actions of others; or, if they do, that it has an impact upon the practice of their colleagues. For example: a teacher who sets out to remedy a discovered gender bias in his mathematics teaching may come to realise the sexist nature of the school text, but may find that there is no money available to replace it; encouraging children to display independence and critical judgement in one's own classroom may alienate colleagues with whom those children also interact; solving a shortage of computers by staggering breaktimes may involve changing a school policy which others wish to maintain. As soon as teachers start to become aware of organizational, social and political structures which impinge on their work, they also become aware of the ways in which power is distributed within their professional worlds. They also learn, if they did not already know, that redistribution of power is often more readily accomplished if people act together. It is very difficult for individual teachers, acting alone, to alter anything in their own situations except their own attitudes or behaviour. Even this may prove impossible, if institutional constraints (eg resources, timetabling), the culture of the school, or the nature of a particular pupil sub-culture forces them to act in ways that they wish to abandon or modify. As a result teacher research often has the effect of making those who undertake it more aware of micro-politics and more ready to engage in them.

Sometimes it also affects researchers' social or interpersonal skills, partly by increasing the likelihood that they will see situations from others' perspectives, partly because of the imperative to act which is often embedded in their enquiries. A straightforward example of the latter process is the teacher who, after exploring why it was always the same children who wanted to contribute in his lessons, decided to become a better listener. In the first instance he tried to increase the wait-time he allowed after he had asked a question. This simple action eventually led to a marked change in his relationship with some of his pupils.

The third main area affected by systematic self-study is that of intellectual competencies. By this I mean that teachers who learn how to engage in self-reflective enquiry develop a range of cognitive abilities which are capable of transfer to other situations (even if they are not always so transferred). I accept that this is risky ground into which to venture; psychologists are likely to find my terms vague and lacking in precise referents, the whole area of cognitive transfer is a vexed one and, once again, I can advance no 'proof' that the intellectual capacities to which I shall refer exist or are enhanced by engaging in practitioner research. Nevertheless, I wish to take that risk.

In my view the cognitive abilities which teacher research is capable of developing can be summed up as perception, understanding, and judgement. Each of these depends for its effectiveness upon the possession of easily-accessed experience or knowledge, though by themselves the latter may inhibit the capacity to perceive, understand or judge (Abercrombie, 1960). Abilities similar to these are noted in Schon's 'reflective practitioner' (1983; 1987) and are inherent in what McClelland (1976) describes as "competency". Further refined, they may be seen as the ability to perceive, conceptualise, analyse and understand accurately the complexities of a particular set of circumstances, to decide which parts or aspects require further enquiry, which are susceptible of modification, manipulation or change and by what sort of action, and which are best left alone because they lie beyond the scope of an individual's or a group's power to alter them. Such capacities involve: seeing, hearing and sensing as full a range of information as possible and processing this in ways that discriminate between salient and irrelevant cues and distinguish between 'fact', value, judgement and inference (for experienced and successful practitioners, this may mean re-learning how to observe); understanding the range of people, events, circumstances which are directly or indirectly involved in a given situation, the likely connections between them and the ways in which change in one may affect the others; discarding, while still retaining the capacity to recall, information which is judged irrelevant; analysing these complexities in appropriate ways; pinpointing those parts of the total situation which seem most salient and those into which further enquiry is most likely to be productive; deciding what action one is likely to be able to take; having a range of alternative strategies on which to draw in selecting appropriate actions; knowing one's own beliefs, biases, abilities, strengths, weaknesses (this points to the importance of autobiographical study).

The notion that teacher research has the potential to develop generalised intellectual competences in its practitioners, leads me to a further point. It is, I think, these or similar capacities which Elliott (1989a, b) has in mind when he speaks of action research developing "practical wisdom, ie. the capacity to discern the right course of action when confronted with particular, complex and problematic states of affairs." His definition draws our attention to the fact that practitioner research is not a technical activity. Discerning the "right" course of action requires moral or philosophical judgements, and therefore knowledge. Education is a "moral science" (Elliott 1989b); research in this field, especially when it is conducted by practitioners, must be defensible by reference to moral criteria or it will not be helping to realise the ends towards which education is directed. Logically, therefore, teacher research must be concerned with the study of ends and not just of means. It follows that philosophers have as large a part to play as social scientists in helping teachers to find a professional voice.

Another way of expressing the notion that systematic school based research can develop particular cognitive abilities is to say that it is governed by "principles of procedure" (Peters, 1966), ie. whatever the topic to be researched, the process of enquiry will be conducted in accordance not with rules but with specified ways of thinking and behaving. In the case of teacher research, these might be described as: all enquiries will arise from the researcher's desire to know more, understand better and improve practice; all situations, practices and understandings chosen for enquiry, and the values underlying them, will be treated as problematic (ie. there are no 'givens', nothing about which questions cannot be asked); the topic or area to be researched will be approached in a synthetic or holistic way; analysis and the use of theory will grow out of, not pre-determine, the progress of the research; every attempt will be made to ensure validity and reliability at all stages. To these principles, many people would add one more: at every stage, the researcher's colleagues and, wherever possible, clients (eg. parents, pupils) will be participants in the research. Since I have already suggested that it is a matter for debate whether collaboration should be seen as logically or pragmatically necessary to practitioner research, I have added it separately, while accepting its importance in practical terms.

In the course of using these "principles of procedure" teachers often internalise them, employing them in other contexts to guide their perception and understanding of situations and their choice of appropriate forms of action. I have observed that ex-students from our courses often seem to become more skilled professionals and problem-solvers, even though they do not continue to engage formally in research. Undertaking school-based enquiry does, over time, seem to assist in the development of professionally relevant intellectual competencies.

Indeed, for some teacher-researchers the two roles become one; the capacities and qualities of skilled researchers are also those which help people to be skilled teachers, and vice versa. Good professional practice (ie. that which promotes educational ends for pupils) is, as Stenhouse (1975) pointed out, a research process, a continual cycle of observation, enquiry, critical reflection and action. Good teaching is research; research promotes good teaching.

However, conducting research in one's own institution and even sometimes in one's own classroom is a delicate social process, particularly since one has to go on living and working with people on whose attitudes or activities one's enquiry may deliberately or incidentally reflect in critical ways. Under these circumstances it is easier to separate one's teacher self from the researcher, to act as a researcher, rather than be a researcher. This is particularly the case for those practitioners who for one or more reasons are isolated within a traditional craft culture. They may lack interested colleagues, they may be loners or may need help in developing collaborative skills, the structures of the school may make it difficult for staff to work together. Whatever the reason, it is understandable that they should choose not to identify too closely with a research process which their colleagues find threatening and alien because it substitutes openness, critical reflection and a willingness to change for the established values of self-reliance, territoriality and respect for established authority.

Yet practitioners who choose to segregate their research from their professional activity (by, for example, formalising and depersonalising data collection methods, Elliott, 1989a) do not, I suggest, learn from the process in the same way as do those who are prepared to face and live with the dilemmas and conflicts which arise from accepting that the interests of the teacher are sometimes at odds with those of the researcher. In other words, practitioner research may involve internal as well as institutional tension. However enriching, it is not an activity for the faint-hearted.

Pedagogue-practitioner partnership

To end this chapter, I wish briefly to comment upon the possible development of a further partnership between pedagogues and practitioners. First, if the two groups are to come even closer together, everyone must feel that they have something to gain from this development. However, the advantages of becoming teacher researchers are so far clear only to a minority of teachers, that is to those who find that combining the roles helps them to be more professionally effective or who derive reflected glory from their association with institutions of higher education. Yet even they have to weigh the benefits of their involvement in practitioner research against the potential threat which their activities and changes in attitude often offer to their colleagues. In practice, many are inhibited by the knowledge that the balance of advantage will frequently tilt against them. Until the dominant culture of teaching alters, this is likely to remain the case. Ironically, in England the introduction of a national curriculum and national assessment, carrying with them as they do the need for staff to talk to one another and to share their expertise, may do more to change this culture than the impact of scattered groups of teacher-researchers.

The association of teacher research with higher education may also play a part in limiting its spread. It is unlikely that the "principles of procedure" implicit in teacher research will be adopted by the majority of the profession until the latter have had the opportunity to make them their own. This can come about only through a much more grassroots approach to practitioner research than currently exists in many schools. If and when this happens, pedagogues may have to accept an altered and diminished role in the partnership. They are also likely to find that many of the conventional indicators of 'research' are changed (in particular, the form and language in which it is presented).

Such a development is beset with dilemmas. If the nature of research is seen to change, some academics may become unwilling to enter into active partnership with the schools. Similarly, if practitioners take control of their own enquiries, some pedagogues may cease to recognise their activities as 'research'. A Catch-22 situation appears to exist. As long as teacher research is directly or indirectly controlled by academics, it will not be widely adopted by teachers. If it is controlled by teachers, it may lose public legitimacy and academic support. The only way forward appears to lie in individuals' willingness to experiment and to sustain any dialogue which may result.

What are academics, for their part, likely to get out of their new relationship with schools, and what may happen if this changes still further? At one level, I and my colleagues get employment – we can 'sell' research expertise and inculcate habits of critical enquiry, reflection and action in the teachers who come on our courses or who seek our services. Much more important is our sense of being closer to the action than we were when we dealt in 'pure' rather than 'applied' research. I greatly enjoy the feeling of involvement, albeit vicarious, in classrooms and schools which results from helping teachers to address in effective ways the issues that are important to them; and I relish the fact that I am close to the cutting edge of educational change, sometimes even sharpening the blades which are used to cut through orthodoxy, preconception or prejudice. Yet I realise that if and when teacher research becomes more institutionalized in schools and alters to accommodate a larger number of practitioners, I shall become further removed from it. And I am not sure how I shall feel if I find myself "training the trainers", deprived of a direct hand in the work of teachers who are struggling to understand and modify their own behaviour and their own situations.

My second point leads on from this and points up another dilemma which is inherent in the relationship between academics and teachers. At present in England (and in many other countries where teacher research is well-established) practitioners are usually given the opportunity to acquire the appropriate expertise through attendance at award-bearing courses (eg. Advanced Diplomas, higher degrees). Many teachers appear to like this arrangement. Most of them have to study part-time; course attendance provides a purpose, a discipline and a structure which it would be difficult to achieve in any other way. Furthermore, such courses also introduce them to research methods and to theoretical approaches which they might lack the motivation to seek out for themselves or of which they might otherwise remain in ignorance. Finally, and crucially, the existence of a group which meets regularly with a common purpose provides its members with the opportunity and usually the obligation to share their attempts at school-based, practice-focussed research. In the process they can experience for themselves the potential and problems of collaborative self-study. Few practitioners would be able to find the necessary time or commitment for such study if the effort were not also linked to regular attendance and the acquisition of a professionally recognised award.

Yet the very existence of such courses and awards is a reminder of academic hegemony. Plainly put, the dilemma is therefore this: Courses run by academics appear to offer the best available opportunity and structure for teachers to learn to become researchers. Yet the existence of, and for course members compulsory attendance at, such courses may encourage both academics and practitioners to maintain their traditional roles in relation to one another.

There are two other related issues. One I have already discussed – the possibility that a new alliance between a minority of both pedagogues and practitioners may be stimulating and professionally enhancing for its members, but fail to make an impact on the majority cultures of either. The other is that course completion does not by itself guarantee the acquisition of attitudes on which the improvement of practice through reflective enquiry ultimately depends. It is possible for practitioners to satisfy all the requirements of a demanding enquiry-based course without this having any apparent long-term impact on their values, understandings or behaviours. Nor does involvement as tutors on such a course guarantee among academics a genuine respect for the practical wisdom and situationally-based expertise of teachers. For the new partnership to succeed each must be prepared to learn from the other. Notwithstanding all of these points I am optimistic. I sense a new spirit among academics and among teachers, and in the course of my work, I am daily made aware of the vigorous and confident voice which English pedagogues are helping their school colleagues to find and sustain. Ironically, it is possible that Thatcherite 'market forces' may strongly contribute to this development. Increasingly, schools can choose whether or not they turn to institutions of higher education for help with professional development. The latter's response is to make their courses and their expertise more accessible to teachers who in turn are often glad of the special strengths which academics can bring to the study of schools and of education. Among these is a knowledge of research and, in this context, of school-based research designed and undertaken by practitioners themselves. Because it is demanding, difficult and sometimes dangerous, and because it runs counter to the traditional culture of schools, teacher research will always be a minority pursuit. Nevertheless this minority is beginning to have a powerful voice. Despite the ambiguities and tensions which it represents, teacher research, itself a synthesis of pedagogic and practitioner expertise, is acting as a yeast within the English educational system. Both as a pedagogue, and as a primary teacher I find it exciting and rewarding to be associated with that leaven. I wish however to maintain its quality and shall continue to do all that I can to ensure that it is characterised by high standards of intellectual integrity and cogent communication. Teacher research must not be de-based through attempts to create for it a spurious mass appeal.

In this chapter, I have outlined the reasons why many teachers find traditional academics both remote and threatening and yet collude with them in maintaining their control of educational theory and research. I have argued that teacher research, despite the criticisms that are made of it, offers a way of renegotiating this relationship, to the benefit of both types of educationalist.

In particular, the process of doing research fosters among teachers the capacity to perceive, to understand and to make judgements from within and about complex practical situations, it increases their interpersonal skills, especially as communicators, and it strengthens their belief in their own efficacy. For their part, academics find that involvement in teacher research, and especially in teaching the courses of which it is an integral component, is challenging, stimulating and profitable work. To be sure, several important dilemmas, relating in particular to the hegemonic nature of research and the forms in which it is made public, remain unresolved. But experiment and dialogue continue and the future looks promising. Pedagogues, assisted by practitioners, are learning to listen and to respond. Practitioners, with the help of pedagogues, are finding a different voice.

Chapter 2

ONLY CONNECT... RELATIONSHIPS BETWEEN HIGHER EDUCATION AND SCHOOLS

Christopher Day, University of Nottingham

The problem

Let us begin by being honest – there is a theory-practice, theoretician-practitioner problem; there is an alienation between those who work in schools and those who work in higher education, between those who are said to practice and those who are said to theorize. Whether we like it or not, this alienation exists partly because of history and partly because of function – after all, how many teachers in schools have time built into their work which allows them to reflect, theorize, research and write? The answer is, of course, very few. However, alienation also exists because many have encouraged this. There is a consciously calculated protective "mystique" surrounding "theory" and "research". This allows one group of educationists to assume power over another. I say, "assume" power because most members of the other group regard "research" and "theory" where they perceive it to be defined as being outside their control as irrelevant to their practical concerns and remote from their practical experience.

Yet no-one denies that value of "finding out more" (researching?) about teaching, learning and the contexts in which they occur. How, then, are these two groups of relative and alienated strangers going to connect? Certainly there will need to be a change in attitudes and relationships. The groups will need to come together much more in co-equal relationships where power, ie. control over knowledge, skills, techniques, is shared and in which the expertise of both groups (the so called theorists and so called practitioners) is valued, seen to be valued, and recognized as being complementary. In a sense (though perhaps not intentionally!) recent legislative changes in England, Holland and elsewhere in Europe, Australia and North America have provided opportunities for new relationships to be formed between higher education and schools. The moves towards the devolution of school budgets and increasing school autonomy as well as accountability have ensured that schools and teachers will engage in more school-centred professional development. For this work to develop assistance will be needed. Otherwise, a new breed of teacher-developers will merely accommodate themselves to the existing norms of the professional craft culture. Teaching may become parochial and insular, unless, at some point, teachers choose to turn to higher education for intellectual, affective and practical support. Table 1 below indicates the dilemmas. If its professional learning assumptions are correct, then external intervention which offers appropriate support and challenge is a necessary condition for extended professional development.

Table 1 The Management of Professional Learning

Professional learning assumptions	External intervention (challenge and support)
Teachers have the capacity to be self-critical	They should be offered the means by which they can begin to engage in deliberative inquiry.
Teachers are motivated to learn by the identification of a problem or issue which concerns professional role (Internal commitment to learning arises out of this).	They should be offered the means to reflect on their thinking and practice (The perceived needs of the clients – the teacher and the school – are of paramount importance in beginning this process).
Effective learning occurs in response to the exploration and confrontation of past and present practice.	Teachers should be offered affective and appropriate moral and critical support in processes of internalization rather than identification or compliance. This support should be provided by peers from their own and other schools and 'critical friends' from other agencies who would work in a partnership with them.
Decisions about change in thinking and practice should arise from reflections on and confrontation of past and present practice.	They should be offered appropriate support in developing strategies for planning; negotiating and implementing work in their own and others' schools.
Transformation in thinking and practice is a necessary part of a teacher's continuing learning process.	Teachers and schools should be supported in the testing or validation of their critical theories through the provision of external consultancy (learning networks, consultants, knowledge brokers)

However, there is a problem here, for not everyone who works in higher education is necessarily able or willing to provide appropriate support. In addition, there is often a "credibility gap" caused by many years of insipid alienation.

My own view is that the alliance between teachers and academics even among those who, like the writers of this book, are committed to developing partnership roles across schools and higher education will always be uneasy. Thus the notion of empowerment of teachers which is so deeply embedded in other chapters of this book; the recognition of a need to develop a new language for communication (eg. Nias) between teachers and academics; and the establishment of self-critical, self-reflecting communities (Handal), whilst attractive, depend for their fulfilment upon the abilities of participants to create contracts, either collectively or individually, which are based on forms of critical friendship.

Critical friendships

Professional development should present opportunities for teachers to escape being prisoners in their own classroom by combining action and reflection. One means of achieving less isolation is through the active encouragement of critical friendships which may be defined as practical partnerships entered voluntarily, based upon a relationship between equals and rooted in a common task or shared concern. They can be a means of establishing links with one or more colleagues from inside or outside the school as well as assisting in processes of learning and change so that ideas, perceptions, values and understandings may be shared through the mutual disclosures of feelings, hopes and fears. Critical friendships can serve to decrease isolation and increase the possibilities of moving through stages of reflection to confrontation of thinking and practice. Reflection in itself will not necessarily lead to self-confrontation, and self-confrontation may need skilled support to be translated into new action. On one's own:

> "one will only see what one is ready to see, one will only learn what is on the edge of the consciousness of what one already knows." (Thompson, 1984)

In terms of the appraisal of classroom practice, for example, a critical friend may establish and sustain a responsive, mutually acceptable dialogue through which situations will be created in which the teacher is obliged to reflect systematically on practice.

The Advantages of Critical Friends (from inside or outside the school) are that, providing they are skilled and trusted, they can:
1. lighten the energy and time loads for observation (enable teacher to carry on teaching, maintain his or her duties);

2. be used to check against bias in self-reporting, and to assist in more lengthy processes of self-evaluation;
3. offer, where appropriate, comparisons with classroom practice elsewhere;
4. move freely and see the curriculum in action;
5. focus in on an agreed issue or area of concern, eg. small group task work;
6. contribute to policy development;
7. act as a resource which teachers, departments and schools may use at times appropriate to the needs which they perceive.

The disadvantages are that if they are unskilled and not trusted then:
1. Unless a regular visitor their interpretations may be out of context. Insiders and outsiders will have their own biases!
2. Teachers may be less open (eg. in interviews).
3. Children and teacher may react to their presence in such a way as to cause untypical behaviour.

Whether teachers invite colleagues from in school or someone from outside (eg. from a local higher education institution) will be a matter for their discretion. However, research suggests that, "It is preferable from the user's point of view to learn from a peer far enough from home so that:
1 asking for help can't be interpreted as a self-indictment;
2. invidious competition and comparison is reduced;
3. the ideas can be challenged with impunity;
4. they can be credited to their new user" (Hopkins, 1986).
Whatever the choice, success depends on:
1. a willingness to share;
2. a recognition that sharing involves:
   (a) disclosure,
   (b) opening oneself to the possibility of feedback;
3. a recognition that disclosure and feedback imply being prepared to consider changing;
4. a recognition that changing is sometimes:
   (a) threatening (to self-esteem and current practice),
   (b) difficult (it requires time, energy, new skills),
   (c) satisfying;
5. a recognition that the degree to which people are willing to share may, therefore, be restricted.
Collegiality, contract making, entitlements and critical friendships are all elements within professional development schemes which support teacher autonomy, and reinforce a sense of responsibility by affirming confidence in teachers' professionalism.

In order to operationalise critical friendships, schools will have to engage in "contracting". This is not intended to be a legalistic process. "Agreements" (a softer, more humane word than contracts) are, of course, often made informally between teachers and increasingly now more formally under "school development plans". Many teachers will have experienced the value of being able to share thoughts, practices and feelings with one or more trusted colleagues. The importance of agreeing contracts is such, however, that it may be necessary to document them for use as aides memoire. Written or at least explicit verbal contracts can do much to clarify mutual expectations as to goals and methods. In other words, the contract needs to be explicit:

- The contract should be negotiated, not proclaimed, by the partners involved.
- The contract should be clear to all involved parties.
- Some kind of oral or written commitment to the contract should be obtained.
- The contract should be reviewed as the parties progress and revised if necessary. (Based on Cormier & Cormier, 1979)

Schon describes this as a "reflective contract", and contrasts it with more traditional agreements:

Traditional Contract	*Reflective Contract*
I put myself into the professional's hands and, in doing this, I gain a sense of security based on faith	I join with the professional in making sense of my case, and in doing this I gain a sense of increased involvement and action
I have the comfort of being in good hands. I need only comply with this advice and all will be well	I can exercise some control over the situation. I am not wholly dependent on information and action that only I can undertake
I am pleased to be served by the best person available	I am pleased to be able to test my judgements about his competence. I enjoy the excitement of discovery about his knowledge, about the phenomena of his practice, and about myself. (Schon, 1983)

In pointing out these differences, he reminds us that the client has the right to make judgements about the "helpers", no matter what role or status they might hold.

Connections in action

The three case study extracts which follow are intended to provide an aperitif for those who wish to develop new partnerships. They are not intended to be models of good practice. But all do provide a linkage between theory and practice; they are client led and client centered; higher education is presented in partnership roles of different kinds. The first describes work in which one teacher was helped to reflect upon his teaching values and practices; the second presents higher education in the role of credible external evaluator to a school-initiated, school-based project involving more than thirty teachers; and the third illustrates higher education in the role of in-service course provider.

case study 1:   working with individual teachers: a client-centered model of researcher intervention (Day, 1985)

The researcher provided the necessary moral, intellectual and resource support for teachers engaged in a process of self-examination – the research was not traditional, for he did not maintain a role distance from the actor and his environment. I believe that by this means the "researcher-consultant" achieved access to more valid information concerning how teachers learn and why they change (or fail to change) – and thus to teachers' thinking – than had he adopted a more neutral or naturalistic stance.

The research set out to test a model of classroom-based in-service education. Members of a secondary school English department volunteered to participate and agreed to the filming of two sequences of six lessons each with fourth-year examination classes. By reviewing these video films and discussing them with the teachers at length, by interviewing pupils and examining the interactions within the lessons, the researcher was able to offer each of the teachers information by which it was possible to re-examine and reflect upon espoused theory and to generate new personal theory. Each teacher's aim was to increase his/her professional effectiveness in the classroom, and five sequential stages were found to be necessary in order to achieve this:

1. Identification of inconsistencies within the prevailing theory of action through self confrontation and reflection;
2. evaluation of this confrontation as a means of informing future decision taking;
3. the planning of new theories-in-use;
4. the implementation of those new theories;
5. internalisation of new theories of action and further confrontation or, return to confrontation of initial theory of action (Day, 1981).

The research was client-centred, in that the researcher intervened in the teacher's life in order to seek questions perceived by the client as relevant to his/her needs; to investigate answers to these questions collaboratively and to place the onus for action on the client him/herself. The notion is that the client's personal investment in the learning enterprise will be maximised. All four teachers involved achieved change at classroom level in different ways, according to their particular intentions. The changes in attitude towards themselves as teachers and towards their teaching were the most significant. Within the constraints of this chapter it is only possible to report briefly on their reactions to their engagement in the process of learning with the support of a researcher, and the changes which they identified in their thinking. Further detail is recorded elsewhere (Day, 1981).

One teacher stated that the work had provided her with the time "to think about, question and even change my methods, and the frame of reference in which to make decisions and formulate ideas." She also stated that one year after the work with the researcher had been completed she still had a more generally questioning attitude as a direct result of the work; and that she had changed as a result of what the study had shown her about herself.

All had already transferred what they had learnt into their work with other classes. The researcher held informal conversations with all the teachers during the two years after the research with them was completed. During the course of these conversations, they often informed the researcher of how the changes they had made in attitude as well as practice were being sustained. They felt that they trusted much more their own ability not only to find, but evaluate and modify their personal solutions to the teaching problems which they encountered. In effect, they felt that they had achieved a new critical standard with regard to themselves as teachers. However, all the teachers commented that without the presence of the researcher, they were unable or unwilling to find the time and energy to continue with the detailed and systematic process of self-evaluation.

In the case of one teacher, Steve, evidence of the long-term changes in thinking was able to be collected both during the supported research process, and at intervals up to five years following its completion. His original goal had been not to allow his teaching to be "dull or unimaginative".

> "What I'm looking for ... is a way of opening up a bit and making things more lively and interesting for them [the pupils] and me, so that I'm better able to get on with them, and the whole experience is more interesting and valuable ..."

He identified a gap between the values held by the school and those held by the members of the English Department – the "norm" for pupils was that the teacher was expert holder of knowledge who viewed the pupils as passive receivers; and what he and the Department valued was "trying to move towards more active participation, more active learning rather than passive learning." However, he was also "torn between wishing for more participation and more liveliness on their (pupils') part, and my consciousness of how much material I want to get through in a given time". He perceived three major constraints:

1. the demands of the examination syllabus for content coverage;
2. the pupils' habits and expectations. They were used to adopting a passive role and tended to be unwilling to change;

3. the pupils' ability. He described many of them as "stodgy", "inert", "fairly passive", and "not particularly able", and he was pessimistic about their ability to progress autonomously and to be fluent in the spoken or written word. He valued self-confidence, humour, and cheerfulness in pupils; and they in turn saw him as "friendly", "encouraging", and "caring" and "helpful".

Steve's planning of his lessons was constrained by his perception that the examination syllabus requirements demanded written work of a particular kind and quantity. These perceived requirements had found expression in the emphasis placed by him on coverage (assimilation) of content selected by him. The result was that he

(a) provided too much for the pupils to assimilate;

(b) made little attempt to discover whether they found the content relevant to their experience;

(c) allowed little deviation in terms of pupil talk from the path leading to his own predetermined conclusions.

In return, the pupils showed their lack of interest by initiating few conversations and by a low level of participation in class discussions. As a result of reflection on his teaching, he succeeded in modifying his organisation, his attitude to content, and his mode of interaction with pupils. He encouraged exploratory pupil talk (Barnes, 1976) through supporting pupils' ideas generally, and not presenting indigestible amounts of pre-selected content. Pupils thus moved from being relatively passive receivers of the teacher's knowledge and opinions and finding answers which were "correct" to being actively involved in the selection and negotiation of content.

Steve's detailed written evaluation of the research contained a clear account of how his attitudes towards it and the researcher had changed:

"... over two years it has progressed from feelings of aloofness, caution and occasional cynicism to ... real professional regard and genuine interest and concern with every aspect of your study – both in your terms and mine ..."

By the end of Steve's first round of research, his commitment to the process was total. In his first written evaluation (a series of chronologically ordered reflections, written three months after our work) he enumerated his thoughts on the value of the process so far:

1. "I was interested in class talk – group talk. The video and tapes helped me to realise what goes on and what doesn't go on behind my back. No other method could show me.

2. I was taught how to ask questions and structure conversations – I hadn't managed to teach myself this in four years. I was taught by seeing my own stultified conversations with kids.

3. I learnt to take it easy in class – not to force all issues and responses into my mould. I got closer to kids too.

4. I found reviewing the video absorbing, reading the transcripts less so. After a while I began to resent spending so much time on it. I began to wonder whether all the time spent was worth what I was gaining. I think it was now – but then I wasn't so sure.

5. Your role – as neutral observer – I accepted and expected. I felt no threat at all, although I was conscious of trying extra hard, being ultra tolerant because there was someone else there.

6. I learnt to revalue the usefulness of resources, particularly teacher produced!

7. It was rewarding to have someone around who had read a lot on our subject and its problems and who could spare the time to have his brains picked over an issue or an author or a book. It helped me take short cuts in thinking about issues like 'talk' or group work or resources because there was someone to bounce half-formed ideas off. Every school should have one."

Steve had become aware of the insecurity of his approach. He wrote:

"...like all teachers I tended to base my approach on a type of paternalism which says, 'Here is what you don't know yet', and I then have the pleasure of whisking back the curtain to reveal...the curriculum...Teachers use the content, the knowledge as a fence between themselves and their group and say, in effect – 'If you want to reach me, as a bloke, you've got to get over the fence first ...'."

He had learnt that he was "creating fences" and he had identified the causes for this as being "the sort of personality I have, by producing pre-selected resources, by pre-figuring class discussions, by asking brief, closed questions, by keeping aloof from the kids ..." He commented on the positive value of self-confrontation and the researcher's role as "consciousness raiser" rather than direct "change agent":

"Your change agency can't change our personalities ... but what I think it can do is reveal to a teacher the nature of his personality in so far as it does or does not elicit responses and promote a learning environment for his group of kids ..."

The first round of research made his implicit theories of action explicit. He then set about re-building these theories in a second round:

"... instead of pre-packaged lessons which bolted on to one another in a pre-ordained way, I tried to let the course build up its own tempo; I took things more slowly, invested time in sometimes lengthy rambling chat full of reminiscence and 'trading' of anecdotes and memoirs. This made me feel happier and more secure with the group as people and probably had a similar effect on them ... Now this seems obvious and basic, but then the most important realisations usually are ..."

I asked Steve if he had felt any positive gain as a result of the research:

"Yes, two. The first one is ... talk, and I allow far more latitude in a constructive way as far as group and individual's talk is concerned. And I try and participate in it more, and steer it more ...

The second thing is, the main gain I think, has been the setting of a higher self-standard, I can't think of any other way in which you'd be so compelled to examine yourself and force yourself as high as you possibly can in the classroom. You try it, and if it works, then you've reached a level to which you must always afterwards aspire, and compare whatever else you do with that. I know when I've fallen short a bit, and I usually know why ..."

Finally, he summarised the value of the research both in terms of its process and product:

"I feel much surer of what the fundamental attributes of a good teacher are in my own mind – without all this navel gazing I would have stayed in my neatly ordered, mechanistic universe for a good while longer. I think I may well have saved myself many errors in approach and the blundering up of a good many blind alleys .. being a part of this research cost me a lot of time and energy. It was worth it ... "

Some five years later, the same teacher wrote about changes that had occurred in his thinking as a result of engaging in the research process. There is little documented evidence of perceived long-term change that has occurred as a result of research or consultancy activities, and so no apology is made for quoting the teacher's unsolicited comments at length:

"My particular concern or perceived need lay in teacher and pupil talk, and it was upon this area that I focused most attention when reviewing the video film of the lessons and in studying tape transcripts. I had prepared a considerable amount of material for discussion, but the talk had not gone well:

'He recognised that not only had he expected pupils to assimilate too much content in too short a time, but that he had demonstrated 'some impatience' ... 'to lead all conclusions my way ...' Indeed his conversations with pupils could be described as games in which the teacher gave the clues (questions) and the pupils searched for correct answers.' (Day, ibid.)

These realisations and others like them grew as the process developed. Having confronted the mis-match between what was and what was desired, the issues were thrown into far sharper focus and it became imperative to abandon the structures I had been relying upon to support 'talk' in my English lessons. In the second sequence I forsook the advance preparation of resources and materials and decided instead to introduce a topic and let the pupils define its direction. The written tasks were self directed and the talk which led up to them I allowed to be steered by the pupils themselves: they were grouped rather than taught as a whole class and I opted to circulate rather than to control from the 'front'.

'Steve's intentions for the second sequence of lessons had been to place more emphasis on

a) developing inter-personal relationships with pupils,

b) giving pupils more freedom to exercise choice in content of work,

c) giving pupils more learning independence from the teacher by adopting an organisational framework dominated by small group and individual work, (

d) modifying his own role from one which tended towards didactic domination of talk to one of facilitating co-respondent in talk (he wanted to talk less, and to ask more questions). In both Steve's view and that of the research, he had gone some way to achieving these changes.' (Day, ibid)

According to Day's evidence, gathered through analysis of all the lesson interactions over the period of several months between the beginning of the first sequence of lessons and the end of the second sequence, the following shifts had occurred.

Class Organisation	Time spent in group work increased, 54% to 77%
Pupil talk in class and group settings (as % of total teacher-pupil talk)	Overall increase from 24-30%; Decrease in class settings from 16% to 11%; Increase in group settings from 31% to 33%
Pupil-initiated conversational incidents with teacher as % of all incidents	Increased from 9% to 33%

Task negotiation by pupils.
Time spent on tasks designated-High/Medium/Low

Major shifts towards high degree of negotiation

0	24	76	Sequence 1
high	medium	low	
61	27	12	Sequence 2
high	medium	low	

Several months later still I wrote an evaluation of the process in which I described what I took to be its important effects: the researcher summarised some of the points I made:

'Steve stated that the self-confrontation process, assisted by the researcher, had taught him to ask questions, structure conversations, value inter-personal relationships in the classroom, re-assess the value and use of teacher produced resources, and re-assess his teaching role. He had undergone a fundamental change of attitude, and a re-adjustment of his self concept. He

believed that his attitude to the process of teaching and learning has changed permanently from 'mechanistic' to 'humanistic'.' (Day, ibid.)
And now:

I can attest to the validity of this model of reflection and theory building. There had been a shift in pedagogy which had come about through the critical evaluation of current practice in the light of both personal and public theory. Close reflection upon practice became an irradicable habit. What is significant, however, is the degree and intensity of external support which was required to engender this. There exists no army of researchers who can institute the process in a wide scale. For me this experience accelerated a process which I hope, but cannot be sure, would have taken place anyway. I was enabled to move out rapidly from my 'comfortable routines' and from the 'coping' strategies which often mark the plateau of many teachers at an early stage in their careers. The process gave me renewed access to public theory in the sense that I could use it: prior to that I was aware of such theory, but could not employ or affirm it because my personal theory was too tightly in the grip of my current classroom practice. By taking a risk and letting go of accustomed practice, by becoming theoryless for a time, I was able to address and assimilate the public theory to which I aspired."

Commensurate to Steve's learning was the researcher's identification of his professional learning theory. The six main principles of it were:

1. effective learning occurs in response to the confrontation of issues by the learner (this reveals discrepancies within and between thought and action);
2. decisions about teaching should stem from reflection on the effects of previous actions (this results in a reassessment of thinking by the teacher about his thinking and behaviour);
3. effective confrontation of issues requires the maximising of valid information (this results in a desire by the teacher to change);
4. video-recordings of lessons provide direct evidence of theories-in-use, and are therefore especially effective in promoting confrontation (which results in attempts to change);
5. effective professional learning requires internal commitment to the process of learning and freedom of choice for the learner;
6. teachers need support in achieving changes – partly because old routines dominate and new routines need support to develop.

Important assumptions underlying these principles are:

a. much knowledge about practice is implicit rather than explicit, so teachers (and indeed researchers) have a limited understanding of theories-in-use;
b. in so far as assumptions about the influence of external factors and the nature of classroom practice remain unquestioned and unproblematic, these are likely to limit a teacher's capacity to evaluate his work;

c. terms such as "reflection" and "informed choice" are taken to imply the need for explicit examination of both espoused theories and theories-in-use;

d. problems in learning new theories of action stem from existing theories which already determine practice, and unless that practice can be related to existing theory explicitly, it is unlikely that any new theories will be developed.

(Detailed evidence for each of these principles can be found in Day, 1979).

In the work described above, since the teacher is seen as an active causal agent in his own learning, the research design cannot be either masterminded or unilaterally controlled by the researcher-consultant. The work must, therefore, be collaborative, with a maximum flow of information between the two and the teacher's and consultant's hypotheses being openly stated as they develop. If this kind of work is to be developed, channels of communication must be established by the research community which enable teachers and researchers to engage in a continuing dialogue about the nature of teaching and learning within the classroom. The active support of an outside agent is necessary:

a. to establish and sustain a responsive, mutually acceptable dialogue about classroom events and their social and psychological context;

b. to audit the process rather than the product of possibly biased self-reporting;

c. to create a situation in which the teacher is obliged to reflect systematically on practice. This is unlikely to happen in the crowded school day;

d. to act as a resource which the teacher may use at times appropriate to the needs which he perceives; eg. to relieve the teacher of the task of data collection;

e. to represent the academic community at the focus of the teacher's professional life. The researcher thus becomes a part of rather than apart from the teacher or client.

Thus a mutually acceptable language of discovery will develop. Problems of transfer (of knowledge), validity and credibility (of research findings) and "barriers to change" will be minimised. In research such as this the two main principles for intervention theory and change are that:

1. the perceived needs of the client(s) are of paramount importance;

2. the consultant's role is collaborative and co-equal, but not necessarily neutral.

Throughout the research, I assumed a model of a teacher who, given particular circumstances, is able to distance himself from the world in which he is an everyday participant and open himself to rational influence by others. I believe that this distancing is an essential first step towards self-evaluation.

Teachers often operate on a model of restricted professionality. Once they have developed a personal solution to any problems of teaching which they perceive – and this is usually achieved without any systematic assistance by others – it is unlikely that this solution will again be significantly questioned. This pattern of teacher development has been characterised as single-loop learning, where theory making and theory testing is private. Argyris & Schon (1976) say about this:

"The traditional researcher also engages in single-loop learning by defining his clients' needs according to what his techniques will allow him to provide. These professional techniques are then reinforced by the institutions which have evolved to make them work (eg. schools and training establishments) and behaviour is constrained to suit them.

Technique thus becomes an instrument of control rather than a means of serving the clients' needs."

Researchers who assist the individual who is attempting to explicate and build his own theory of practice, are, as Steve recognised, engaged in diagnosis (of the world in which he acts), testing (of his theories and assumptions) and the accepting of personal causality (taking responsibility for what he does); and these elements refer both to technical theories (techniques which the practitioner uses in his work) and interpersonal theories which state how the practitioner interacts with his clients during his work.

Though there are now a steadily growing number of researchers who are going into classrooms, they do not always do so with the purpose of supporting teacher learning in the ways outlined here. All too often, they too operate in their world of restricted professionality and, like other professionals, protect themselves and their colleagues by speaking in abstractions without reference to directly observed events. This has the effect of both controlling others and preventing others from influencing oneself by withholding access to valid information about oneself. The time is ripe not only for researchers to get into the classroom where the action is in order to understand it, but for a truly collaborative approach which embodies more open access by the research "subject" to the researcher's thinking and practice to the ultimate benefit of both.

Case study 2:   researcher as evaluator

This case study is based on the researcher's experience in the role of evaluator of a school-based curriculum development scheme located at a large secondary school in England. Over a one year period, five separate projects were undertaken by different groups of teachers on a voluntary basis. The numbers of teachers involved constituted almost half of the total school teaching staff of seventy three. Each group had a leader who was allocated two periods each week off timetable, and the groups themselves were allocated between ten and twenty days to conduct their investigations. The key feature which underpinned the scheme was that:

"teachers themselves can be active in promoting changes of style or content which will lead to significant developments across the curriculum" (Branston, 1986).

This view of teachers as experts represents an assertion of "the creative power inherent in the group of teacher colleagues" in the school (Schmuck and

Schmuck, 1974). The scheme reflected not only particular notions of the ways in which teachers learn and the conditions necessary for learning to occur effectively, but also the belief that there can be no curriculum development without teacher development (Stenhouse, 1975). Significantly, monitoring and evaluation processes were built into the scheme. Traditionally, most of the resources and effort to promote curriculum and teacher development have been concentrated on the initiation and developmental stages themselves, and little, if any, have been devoted to monitoring (ie. the systematic collection of information) and evaluation (ie. making judgements, whether formative or summative, based upon information collected). The scheme avoided this temptation via internal and external monitoring. The external monitor needed to be a sympathetic outsider to tell participants what is happening as they go along.

"People who will really listen as we try to manage our own INSET and school development, and later be able to report our feelings as people, our perceptions as professionals, our achievements as educators ...." (Branston, 1986a).

It is important at this point to define more precisely the role of the external evaluator in this school-based curriculum development work. Clearly, s/he cannot be "the" authority, since every member of every project group is an authority within the teacher-as-expert model. The role is to "objectify" the conditions, purposes, processes and outcomes of the projects by documenting the perceptions, over time, of those who are involved directly and indirectly. In order to achieve an evaluation which is derived from the cultural perspective of the participants, the evaluator has to seek inside information and respect indigenous definitions and values. This kind of evaluation, "tries to define how people see things from within" (House, 1981). It is collaborative rather than hierarchical, relying upon the collection, interpretation and validation (by the participants) of information through documents, observation, and face-to-face interviews. The evaluator must thus establish credibility by encouraging the creation of a climate of openness and trust with each of the individuals with whom he works. Essentially, s/he also has an investment in and commitment to the professional growth of teachers, the improvement of schools in general, and teaching and learning in particular. The assumption here is that outside experts who "know best" cannot easily improve schools and teaching. Indeed:

"This trend in thinking that there surely is someone somewhere who knows best and can decide for one is a form of self-domination that is profoundly ironic (and is) destined to promote infantilisation of teachers rather than secure their growth" (Bell, 1985).

In contradistinction, the criteria for success of this project were:

a. projects should centre on an important school issue (of curriculum or learning styles, and related organisational/struc-tural implications);

b. projects should be collaborative. Participation in them, the process, should be regarded as an important outcome in itself, as a way of supporting the view that school self-analyses and self-renewal are key aspects of a teacher's professionality;

c. projects should lead to, or clearly prepare for, an actual change;

d. project teams should be deliberately and clearly linked to the normal, on-going processes and bodies which in theory "manage" curriculum maintenance and review (eg. Academic Board or Heads of House or Staff Conferences) so that the danger of isolation is avoided, and so that the proposal has maximum status and impact;

e. projects should clearly relate, immediately or less directly, but always, to classroom interactions. The stimulation of direct consideration of, or research into, what happens at the point of learning should be an aim. Teachers should be encouraged to become their own researchers into classroom phenomena (Branston, 1986).

The projects were to be pursued by communities of equals and success would therefore be the result of collaboration.

This case study contains brief descriptions of and comments upon two of the five projects. (A complete report is contained in Day, 1990b). These descriptions are based upon attendance at and documentation of meetings and data gathered through tape recorded interviews with project participants. Following the descriptions of the projects, I wish to discuss the extent to which the criteria already described were met and, in general, consider the nature of teacher learning and change, as well as the management of school based curriculum development.

The two projects

Curriculum Descriptions Group

"All teachers are concerned with the curriculum. It's fundamental to what we do ... What we all do is to close our classroom door and shut the school out ...."

A group of six teachers aimed to produce a "summary of the curriculum offered to Branston pupils, such that all staff could gain some insight into the experiences children were receiving in areas other than personal specialisms" (Williams, 1987).The project was divided into two areas:

(a) discovering what the curriculum is, and how it is delivered;

(b) investigating a means of presenting a description of the whole curriculum in a comparatively immediate and accessible form.

During term one of the project members devised a questionnaire, based upon elements of learning and administered it to all staff who taught first year (11 year old) pupils. The questionnaire format was adopted as being "the most expedient means of soliciting information from a comparatively large number of subject areas" (Williams, 1987). The intention was to discover and describe the framework of the curriculum, what overlap of subject areas and interests, and what complementary material and approaches were present. Despite doubts as to its adequacy the questionnaire results did provide the desired base for analyses and description.

Term two was spent in pupil pursuits in order to "gather a flavour of the curriculum on offer". In this exercise five members of the group observed the same class of first year pupils on each day of the same week in order to gain an overview of the curriculum in action. Five viewpoints were felt to be of value – despite the recognition that there would not be a single conformity of view. Teaching purposes were taken into account, activities in lessons were recorded sequentially and timings were taken. In addition, pupils were interviewed. The results were analysed and discussed and provided the information presented in Terms 1 and 2 of the following year at two separate feedback meetings.

The group reported on issues concerning the curriculum (balance of age and experience of staff; possibilities of gender stereotyping) and the relationships between the ways in which different subject departments "delivered" the curriculum. Some of the findings are illustrated in this excerpt from the final report:

"Far more pupil listening takes place than might normally be supposed – In many subjects far less was anticipated. Less discussion takes place than might be expected. Similarly, far less exercising and developing of reading and writing skills takes place than might have been supposed .... The project raised many pertinent questions, the answers to which cannot but help shape future curriculum planning, for example, what is the comparison between

1. how children learn (best) with
2. how children are expected to learn.

The percentage of time children (should) spend working individually, in pairs, in groups, in classes etc. needs to be researched.... the more staff can observe other staff teaching, and students learning, the more will be the general awareness of what the curriculum really is, and less the need for a description." (Williams, 1987).

Learning about Learning Group (entitled originally "Classroom Phenomena")
The support for this kind of project was fundamental to the belief in teacher-as-expert; and the purposes were described as being:
– to stimulate the teacher-as-researcher/analyst model,
– to emphasise classroom experience as "worthy of primary, personal analysis by teachers themselves, as the obvious and in fact only possible 'experts' in promoting learning" (Branston, 1986).

The most important intended outcome was described as "an increase in confidence among teachers that they can discuss, theorise about and be active in the management of learning (or the environment it happens in) and that they are the natural experts at analysis of its features" (1986, op cit). This coincided with the group's aspirations for a heightened awareness of what they were doing which would "rub off in conversation with other people". None of the group had any previous experience of classroom research. Members had agreed to focus upon classroom interaction; they began by observing their own classrooms, focusing upon areas which were of particular personal interest. The main aim of this was, "to enable us to clarify our ideas about possible fruitful areas of research." These observations were then shared in the group. Impressions recorded at the end of the first term were described as "striking, particularly the 'blinkeredness' and isolation of much pupil experience in the classroom." As a result of discussion, the main areas of interest which emerged were: teacher questioning as an aspect of teacher/student exchanges; and how best to motivate students and encourage them to take greater initiative in their learning. A decision was made to focus first upon the volume and types of teacher questioning through the observation of colleagues' classrooms from within and outside the immediate project group. This was to fulfil the group's agreed secondary aim, "to acquire experience of methods of research, especially of observing each other teaching." An aim which was of equal importance, however, was, "to achieve a greater sense of team identity, greater ease of co-ordinating the group's work and ... being able to meet to discuss common ground."

Below is an extract from the team leader's report on this part of the group's research:

"Six members of the group each observed at least 70 minutes worth of lessons, recording the types of questions used by teachers on an analysis sheet ..... The strongest impression formed by the group was of the sheer number of questions generated by teachers. This surprised both the observers and the observed. The most startling case involved a teacher who had been happy to have a lesson of hers observed, though rather apologetic that the lesson would not involve many questions; in fact 110 were recorded in 35 minutes ....

Observers were left with the impression that rather too often questions were just a method teachers had of controlling or dominating a discussion; rather than provoking thought they could in fact dull the student's receptiveness to the occasional really valuable question." (Laycock, 1988).

Whilst seasoned researchers from outside schools will find little to surprise them in this information it is worthwhile emphasising that many of the teachers were learning this for themselves for the first time and were deeply affected by their discoveries.

As a result of these discoveries, the group decided to try to view the experienced curriculum from the pupils' viewpoint. Five members engaged in student pursuits each following a different student from the same mixed ability first year class (11-12 year olds) through a day's lessons on different days of the week. They reported that:

"We had come a long way since the group's first tentative exercises in observing fellow group members. Two factors may have been particularly important in ensuring the success of the exercise: we were seen to be a reasonable cross-section of ... teachers directing our own research; and, furthermore, our emphasis was now on observing students and learning rather than teachers and teaching."

Clearly this was a group which grew in confidence through the year. The final report reflected this and the learning which occurred from the student pursuits:

"One of the strongest impressions to emerge from this section of our research was of how isolated many of the students seemed to be – from their teachers and from their peers. A well motivated and academically able girl whom we observed even managed to remain unaware of the excitement caused in a science lesson by a minor fire in another part of the laboratory. Perhaps more interesting, however, was that her periods of deep concentration would be broken regularly – typically about every twelve minutes – by a pause for taking stock or simply relaxing. During the science lesson already mentioned, for example, she left her table ostensibly to fetch some apparatus but in fact simply to be able to wander round and look out of the window. In a remarkably sophisticated way her learning was already largely self-directed. This girl was in many ways exceptional but for different reasons the activities of peers and teachers seemed to have very little impact on at least two of the other students to be observed, boys of average and weak academic ability. One member of staff commented on the latter that school was a phenomenon in his universe that wouldn't hurt him if he didn't hurt it. In this context it seemed significant that observers commented on the very small amounts of time when students were expected to produce or discuss work in groups."

This work led the teachers to investigate group work as a means of countering the sense of isolation noted in the student pursuits.

Management of school-based curriculum and professional development
The issues in the management of school-based curriculum and professional development which emerged, centered on the external evaluator's role. I was supposed to help future development not only by providing feedback to, "people starting off on something new, having only a partial glimpse of what other people have done ..." but also through an evaluation report which would seek to place the

work and views of their members in a broader explanatory framework. There are a number of specific and general issues which arise from the scheme which may be useful for both action participants and managers in furthering knowledge about the planning, process and outcomes of school-based curriculum development.

The first issue concerns the question: "Does the use of action research in school-based curriculum development lead to emancipation or control?" In keeping with the projects notion of "teacher-as-expert" there was an assumption that the teachers in these projects already possessed a great deal of knowledge and understanding of the contexts which they were going, to investigate – "People are going into this with what they've already learned as chalk face practitioners" but that through the systematic analysis of a specific aspect of school life, they could begin to articulate the principles underlying practices more clearly and so "present them for critical self-scrutiny and for examination by colleagues" (Nixon, 1987). Essentially, the projects gave the participants the opportunity to move from a normal mode of "insider activity" (Ebbutt, 1982) in which they worked in their own classrooms, reflected on their own practice from time to time, incorporated the results of their reflections into their practice sometimes, but did not collect data systematically nor produce written reports, towards a teacher researcher "classic" action research mode. Here the teachers worked in their own (and sometimes other) classrooms as part of a coherent group which met regularly. They systematically collected and analysed data concerning their own and colleagues practice, generated hypotheses and wrote reports open to public critique. In addition (the dissemination phase) they worked towards improvement by testing hypotheses at institutional level. In this very real sense they were involved in innovation and change, promoting confrontation of thinking and practice at both personal and institutional levels. It is necessary, therefore, to view this school-based curriculum development work against a backcloth of the innovation and change model which underpinned the projects:

1. Teachers were active participants in research which contributed to "the practical concerns of people in an immediately problematic situation" (Rapaport, 1970). The process had begun as a result of a feeling of dissatisfaction by the Principal with certain aspects of school life and these feelings were shared, in most cases, by those who participated voluntarily in the projects.
2. A key feature of the research was that "team members themselves take part directly or indirectly in implementing the research" (Cohen and Manion, 1980).
3. In particular the focus of each project had "deep personal significance" (Shumsky, 1958) for the teacher-researchers involved.
4. The projects developed in the classic action research manner, beginning with the "felt need" through planning a practical response or "strategic action" (Grundy, 1983), to the implementation of what has been described as "small scale intervention in the functioning of the real world" (Cohen and Manion,

1980), and the concurrent formative evaluations of this, to, finally, retrospective reflection through which the participants may adopt new thinking and/or practice or have those which are currently held reinforced. (These processes will have begun during the action research itself.) In short, action research informs practice.

But this raises an important issue for those who seek or are offered resource support for action research work; for inevitably there will be an institutional needs dimension which will have to be taken into account and may conflict with the personal or group needs dimension. In any need identification procedures and staff and curriculum development programmes, this matching between felt individual and institutional need is bound to be potentially problematic. Much attention, particularly in England (Elliott, 1980; Simons, 1979; Day, 1981) and also Australia (Kemmis et al 1981; Smyth, 1987) has been given to establishing a particular ethical framework for the control of action research, so that, for example, "involvement should be voluntary and teachers should retain a high degree of control over the direction of the action research and the confidentiality surrounding their contributions" (Wallace, 1987). In this conception the primary focus is upon groups of teachers using action research frameworks (practical and ethical) to support the improvement of their own practice. Kemmis (1981) has distinguished between "practical" and "emancipatory" action research:

"Action research .... can be practical (ie. deliberate groups decide the best ways to act within existing constraints) or emancipatory (the process of reflection leads to action based upon a critique of the social milieu). Just as the patient is emancipated from the oppression of his psyche through the process of self-reflection, so also in social theory, the act of self-reflection within critical communities is emancipatory .... The emancipation of participants in the action .... from the dictates or compulsions of tradition, precedent, habit, coercion, or self-deception."

Whilst the process of action research which occurred in the project groups was emancipatory in the sense that their participants were free to opt in, design and implement, and evaluate, the emancipation of the mind and spirit did not always lead to empowerment in terms of the ability to change individual and collective practices and policies. Work undertaken which attempts to support curriculum and staff development through teacher research, runs the risk of being seen as an instrument of control rather than empowerment when the research is prescribed by curriculum needs or policies defined by an individual or group of staff who hold senior positions within the management structure of an institution.

In summary, what have I learned which may help in promoting more effective and efficient teaching and learning? This summary of issues derived from the experiences of the participants and those of the evaluator are presented in the form of propositions for establishing and developing effective school-based curriculum development work:

1. Curriculum Development as the Servant of Continuing Professional Development:

   Research in teaching and curriculum development are integral to professional development. Curriculum research and reform should be viewed as activities which serve the needs of professional development rather than vice-versa. School-based developments must be continuing rather than sporadic.

2. Motivation, Commitment and Ownership:

   Tension between individual, school and externally identified needs must be recognised. Whoever initiates an idea, it is crucial that those involved in pursuing it are, and perceive that they are, able to adapt and adopt so that it ultimately belongs to them. If this is recognised and acted upon will, motivation and commitment are likely to be achieved.

3. Collaborative Planning:

   A hallmark of successful development is the extent to which there is shared decision-making between teachers and management and teachers who work in the same team.

4. Contracting and Team Building:

   Teams must be given the power to make decisions and to participate fully in the planning, processes and evaluations of their work. The parameters for decision-making must be negotiated initially and, where appropriate, renegotiated. Programmes must be available which enable team leadership and team building skills to be acquired.

5. Voluntarism:

   Voluntarism is a basis for action rooted in faith and personal feeling. It is developed through dialogue and thought and is a sine qua non for successful professional and curriculum development.

6. Reflection, Analysis and Participation:

   Learners must be active participants in their own learning. Successful professional development is that which assumes that the experiences and intuitions of practitioners are of prime value. It consciously employs reflection, analysis and experimentation by providing active opportunities for participants to move from intuition to the disciplined collection of experiential knowledge. In this way the records of vicarious experiences may lead to further experiential and propositional knowledge.

7. Horizontal Relationships:

   Relationships are likely to be more effective when based upon the notion of "professional community" rather than "hierarchical direction". Lateral rather than hierarchical structures within organisations will be more effective. Peer groups are the best bases of influence.

8. Problem Identification and Individualism:

   No two departments or schools are exactly alike. Therefore the judgements made about curriculum and action made by those in them must not lightly be supplemented, ignored or dismissed. Problem identification must be both systematic and situation specific.

9. The Use of Human Resources:

   There should be a prime but not exclusive reliance on the use of internal rather than external human resources (ref. Proposition 6).

10. Support of Management:

    Institutional support of a material and psychological – moral kind is essential in order to provide time, energy, a sense of task and teacher being valued, and a mutually acceptable time-frame. Planning must take account of the need for interim adjustments in the kinds and levels of support to take account of individual affective factors (eg. fatigue, lessening of commitment).

11. Knowledge Dissemination and Utilization:

    Decisions concerned with the dissemination and utilization of knowledge outside the individual participant or participant group must be made at the planning stage and appropriate support built into the processes of any professional and curriculum development scheme. To be effective, dissemination must be founded upon principles of ownership, negotiation, collaboration and shared decision-making. It may be enough that scheme participants themselves have gained from their involvement. Dissemination must be recognised as a complex process which may be inappropriate in this kind of work.

12. Harmony:

    An underlying variable which is critical for effective implementation of structural and procedural change is teacher-principal harmony:

    "Working relations between administrators and teachers had to be clear and supportive enough that the pressures and stresses of incorporating something new could be managed together. The message of our own model is that both teacher mastery/commitment and administrative action are critical for institutionalisation – and that linkage between them can be achieved." (Miles, 1983)

Case study 3: higher education as in-service consultant (Day, 1990a)

This case study illustrates the way in which, through initial contracting, negotiation, and a mix of off- and on-site peer-assisted work over a period of nine months, forty teachers engaged in processes of professional learning and change which affected themselves and their schools. It raises issues of professional intervention through consultancy and provides evidence through independent evaluation, observation and personal testimony which supports the notion of effective professional and institutional development through a mixed economy of professional opportunities for teachers in collaboration with outside agencies. The course which will be described was collaboratively planned, and based upon a recognition that the most important teaching and learning resource is the teacher him/herself. It extended over a period of ten working days between June and March, and was divided in six related phases:

June	Phase 1	Contracting (half-day attended by heads and curriculum leaders)
June – September	Phase 2	School-based peer-supported classroom observation task (half-day)
September	Phase 3	First residential phase (three days)
September – February	Phase 4	School-based peer-supported negotiated curriculum development (two-and-a-half days)
March	Phase 5	Second residential phase (three days)
June	Phase 6	Networking continued (locally negotiated meetings)

The need for the course was identified initially by a consultative committee on which the teaching profession, higher education and local education authority advisory and inspection services were represented. A half-day seminar was held to which curriculum leaders (defined as teachers in schools with designated responsibility for the development of one or more aspects of the curriculum) were invited. Here, specific needs and preferred learning models were identified. A planning team of inspectors/advisers and teachers chaired by a higher education colleague was formed which, preceding the launch of the course, determined the philosophy, structures, practices and resources for the course.

The planning group meetings themselves were in fact a form of collaborative professional development, since all the members did not know each other, many had different viewpoints and experiences (eg. in large or small schools, urban or rural) and they had not all been involved in course design before. It is crucial that the course director/convener is able to ensure that the group becomes cohesive and coherent as soon as possible. Just as important, the course planning enterprise must establish corporate responsibility in practice. The experience of this writer suggests that effective planning will only emerge from a mutually supportive consultancy exercise in which the model of learning matches that intended for the course itself. The course aimed to help its members "become more effective curriculum leaders, have improved knowledge and skills of leadership, and be better able to lead and be part of a team; to become more aware of current educational thinking, and be able to plan, support and evaluate curriculum development in conjunction with their headteacher and colleagues." The central theme of the course was the role of the curriculum leader and from this arose three related topics:

a. leadership: helping qualities and skills;
b. working alongside colleagues in professional and curriculum development in the classroom and in the staffroom;
c. observing teachers and children in the classroom.

In addition to the course content work, members were required to undertake pre-course and interphase tasks which, would "be of practical relevance to their roles as curriculum leaders and their work in their own schools."

The residential phases and their contents were built around the school-based work, and the initial contracting that had taken place. The dominant mode of organization was small group work in which participants shared experiences and opinions critically; and "pairings" of participants in order to provide "close" support for school-based work. The small group work was complemented by "expert" input on issues related to the management of curriculum and professional development, and local group networking. This reflected the planners desire to minimize or avoid problems of knowledge transfer and ownership which are often associated with the more traditional patterns of in-service training, while at the same time avoiding the problem of parochialism which is associated with school-based work. The course was, in effect, an extended exercise in consultant supported school-focused development. It was designed specifically to enable teachers to reflect systematically on their thinking and practices and to provide active support for teachers in their learning processes and in the planning, implementation and evaluation of changes.

The first step was to introduce and actively encourage the notion of contract making:

1. *with self*: to undertake to give the commitment, time and resources in order to fulfil obligations as a professional;
2. *with school*: to ensure that colleagues in school benefit from my attendance on the course through regular feedback;
3. *with course members*: to agree with colleagues on the course to build trust through willingness to share and receive feedback; and to provide moral, intellectual and practical support as appropriate;
4. *with course organizers*: to attend all sessions; to fulfil written work requirements and to share these within negotiated frameworks of confidentiality; to contribute expertise and experience in small and whole group work;
5. *with L.E.A.*: to ensure that the L.E.A. benefits from my attendance on the course through affirmation/enhancement of my current management practices in school; and to be prepared to contribute to L.E.A. in-service work where appropriate and through negotiation.

It was not expected that contracts or agreements would be completed immediately – indeed, quite the reverse, since in many cases staff would have to be consulted. It was recognized also that for many the idea of written agreements is alien, since the predominant primary school culture is that of informality, trust and collaboration. However, although there was no compulsion, most did make a written agreement. The comments below express the range of response to the task:

> "I came away feeling bewildered ... when it came to writing the contract we both found it very difficult ... I don't think my head and I really needed a contract as I know she would support me wherever possible ... it must be left to the teacher and head to work out for themselves if they need a contract ..."

> "I've never made a written contract before but can really see the value of them. They are: good for setting targets; good for negotiating time for task; good for ensuring commitment."

> "The rock on which the whole thing (task) has been built has been the contract made first with Head and then with colleagues in my own school. We would have gone nowhere slowly without these."

The residential phases of the course were intended to build on the contracting by providing opportunities for teachers to distance themselves from the classroom in order to reflect on and plan for action in a variety of ways. The curriculum of these phases was in part prescribed (in relation to the advertised content of the course), in part self-generated (through school-based issues) and in part negotiated (through the peer group challenge and support groups which acted as reference points and met throughout the year). The task was to, "plan and implement or evaluate/monitor a small-scale piece of curriculum development with one or more colleagues in your own school, including classroom observation. This should take account of the developmental context of your school, but not be dictated by it. The task is to be documented and shared with colleagues during the second residential phase." The emphasis upon school-based work is important, since it underlined the planners' subscription to the "practicality ethic" of teachers. Course members would value the work if they perceived it as having direct and tangible practical benefits for themselves and their schools. It was assumed that moral and practical support would be necessary, so this was built into the work through peer pairing and network support groups.

In summary, it is clear, then, that the course was designed specifically to enable teachers to reflect systematically on and confront their thinking and practices; and to provide active support for them both in their learning processes and in the planning, implementation and evaluation of curriculum development in school. This arose through the school-based action research which, with the learning networks, formed the central core of the course. Deliberative reflection and inquiry, contracting (with self and others), self- and peer-confrontation, and the sharing of insights gained from this are posited as essential ingredients in professional learning. The reflective responses of the course members were documented in course diaries to which only the writer had access, and an independently conducted evaluation report was conducted.

Most members found that the classroom observation task (Phase 2) was "for their own benefit" but "has led to a general interest amongst staff in observations." In fact:

"Course members seemed to find this task of benefit to themselves and also to their schools. Many indicated that they had learned or developed generalised skills such as co-operation with colleagues, how to gain access to colleagues classrooms, the value of staff meetings and how to lead. There was also a sense that people felt more valued for their leadership qualities and that colleagues did take them more seriously. The awareness of the needs of colleagues also appeared to be heightened by the task including the value of listening to others, using their suggestions and a realisation that staff do welcome help." (Banks 1988).

All the diaries reflected this valuing of the opportunity to engage in an extended piece of curriculum and professional development that had been "legitimized" through course and contracts:

"Other members of staff are beginning to take an interest in the work we are doing. Teachers are beginning to stop me and ask advice on an informal basis ... I am beginning to appreciate the skills of the other members of staff I am working with."

The evaluator had asked course members to comment on how the course had affected:

(a) their competence and effectiveness as curriculum leaders;

(b) their knowledge and skills for leadership;

(c) their ability to lead and be part of a team;

(d) their general awareness of current educational thinking; and

(e) their ability to plan, support and evaluate curriculum development with their headteacher and colleagues.

All of these areas had figured in the purposes and intended outcomes sections of the course. The evaluation reports stated that:

"From the responses it was evident that everyone felt that they had increased their competence and confidence in most, if not all of these areas. The sense of improvement in self-esteem and confidence was particularly striking." (Banks, 1988).

Teachers attending professional development activities will be in different "states of readiness" to engage in learning – even where they themselves have participated in the planning. They will have different specific needs since they are likely to be at different stages in their own personal and professional develop-ment. Moreover, there can be no assumption that all the participants will be operating with equal effectiveness in their different school contexts. This will depend upon life and professional life cycle factors as well as those which are associated with the school culture.

The assumption both in the planning and processes of the course was that professional development cannot be forced. Teachers cannot be developed (passively), but can best develop (actively). The problem is that although much teacher learning occurs naturally, gradually and by a variety of means, so much of this growth is unnoticed (by those outside the school), many changes are slow and unperceived (often even by the teacher); and growth in learning is not linear. With this in mind, the planners attempted through course structures and processes to:

1. *Support and extend teachers' capacities to be self-critical*

   Although most teachers are capable of reflecting on their thinking and practice, few have the time or energy to do this systematically or deliberatively. The quality of the teachers reflective framework is a decisive factor in his or her development and that opportunities for the growth of clarity and awareness of ones own thinking and behaviour must therefore be built in as essential items to this course. The teachers themselves, then, acted as researchers (Stenhouse, 1975) within an action research model which involved conscious reflection and "consciousness raising" through dialogue provided by course tutors, peers and invited lecturers/workshop leaders.

2. *Ensure participation in and ownership of the learning*

   Since most teachers share needs of: affiliation – the need for a sense of belonging (to a team); – achievement – the need for a sense of "getting some-where" in what is done; appreciation – the need for a sense of being appreciated for the efforts one makes; influence – the need for a sense of having some influence over what happens within the work setting; ownership – the need for a sense of personal investment in the process of curriculum development and its outcomes, it was hypothesized that teachers would give serious consideration to findings which they themselves had made, and that in this way their understandings and perceptions of their work would be enhanced. This model of learning asserts that connections between thinking, learning and actions arc both acquired and made explicit through self-generated work, which is perceived as relevant and appropriate by each individual teacher.

3. *Support of self and peer confrontation of problems or issues*

   Private assumptions as well as practices must be shared, and opened up for questioning (by self and scrutiny by others). Therefore, the process of development is unlikely always to be comfortable – even where extensive negotiations have taken place, contracts made and forms of confidentiality ensured. Consciously suspending judgements about ones own work will almost inevitably raise doubts about what under ordinary circumstances appears to be effective or wise practice. Yet the raising of doubts is only the first in what will be a number of potentially painful steps along the road to change – a road which can be littered with obstacles of time, energy, resources and, perhaps most important, self doubt.

The individual programme of professional and curriculum development was therefore strengthened by peer support which was built into the course structure and processes. Teachers were thus enabled to confront their beliefs in the light of new personal and practical knowledge; reflection and confrontation were seen as a necessary prelude to transformation. *To achieve this it is necessary to set up channels of communication through in-service courses which enable teachers and consultants to engage in a continuing dialogue about the nature of teaching and learning within agreed contexts.*

Where I refer to consulting or consultant, I intend, like Steele (1975), the emphasis to be on a particular process, not on a strict occupational role:

> By the consulting process, I mean any form of providing help on the content, process or structure of a task or series of tasks, where the consultant is not actually responsible for doing the task* (*Anything a person, group or organisation is trying to do.) itself but is helping those who are. The two critical aspects are that help is being given, and that the helper is not directly responsible within the system (a group, organisation or family) for what is produced. Using this definition, consulting is a function, not an occupational role per se. (Steele, 1975)

Within this consulting process, the kinds and timings of interventions which are made are critical. The building of trust and credibility, and affective support provided by the consultant are paramount. As consultant I had a Teacher role (Knowledge broker): "...At times my main function has been simply to teach ... I use didactic processes, such as seminars ... but ... I am defined as the teacher and clients are students..." I was course talisman wherein my presence provided a sense of security and legitimacy allowing the client to feel comfortable enough to experiment in areas where he might not act without support. Furthermore, I had a "shot-in-the-arm role" as sympathetic outsider. I provided added legitimization and moral support. This moral support was particularly important as the project developed, when some teachers felt "negative effects of innovation", eg. an increase in work load/anxiety. There is also the Clock role/collector task:

> "There have been projects where my most important role seemed to be that of a timer or clock for the client system to watch. My presence (or the thought of it coming soon) served as a spur to clients to be thinking and experimenting so that they would have something to show me for the time in between my visits" (Steele, 1975).

It had been negotiated that teachers keep diaries and that the school-based tasks be documented: I was seen as "collector" in fulfilment of a properly negotiated initial contract.

I stress that there is a need for the consultant to establish from the beginning a "private" relationship with each client as a basis for building confidence and trust, so that, for example the individual client or client group will know that whatever is said and whatever information is collected will be under his/her control. (Will anyone else see the videotapes of classroom teaching or the report of the school? If so, who, and at what stage?) Care must be taken that those who deliberately place themselves in a "vulnerable" position where their work may be subject to judgement by unknown (or even known) others are reassured of the confidentiality of the material. "Action research cannot be undertaken properly in the absence of trust established by fidelity to a mutually agreed ethical framework governing the collection, use and release of data" (Elliott, 1978).

Many programmes of professional development are based on what I believe to be a myth – that one can simply sit down with others, work out aims et cetera and implement them. They do not take into account such concerns as anxiety, status and identity (Hoyle, 1970). In work which is concerned with a questioning of the teachers self-image, the affective area is rarely made explicit in the documentation of professional development work. Yet, it is clearly crucial for the in-service educator to consider the attitudes of the teacher, not only to the process of innovation, but also to the interventionist role of the consultant which is part of that process. How does the teacher perceive the consultant? Is he an authority or a threat? Is he a process helper or a judge with alien values?

The partnership model presented here may be translated into different kinds of in-service events at different levels. The final part of this chapter will focus on the contexts in which the management of professional learning occurs.

What I have concluded from this research is in support of a mixed economy in in-service education. For some years now there has been a continuing debate concerning the relative effectiveness and efficiency of different forms of professional development opportunities for teachers. This debate has centred implicitly upon notions of purpose, ownership, relevance and utilization. Whilst all would agree that the ultimate purpose of in-service work is to enhance the quality of education for pupils, the means by which this purpose is best achieved most effectively and efficiently are in dispute – hence the variety of activities, courses and conferences. Traditional, off-site professional development in the form of secondments to institutions of higher education has been criticized because these seem to have benefited the individual more than the school. School-based in-service – the other end of the continuum – has itself been criticized because of its parochialism (Henderson and Perry, 1981). The central issues in both kinds of extreme have been need identification, ownership, application, relevance and, implicitly, "value for money" (interpreted as accountability to employers).

Increasingly, the argument has been made that, with limited financial resources available, professional development opportunities can only be supported centrally where they can be seen to relate directly to the needs identified by national or local government and schools. The net effect of this is that there has been a growth in school-based work and short courses designed for particular pupuses and a decline in full-time students registering for courses in institutions of higher education. In those areas where there is a tradition of collaboration between higher education, schools and LEAs (which, for example, involves joint planning meetings to design in-service work, needs identification groups consisting of LEA, schools and higher education representatives, visits to schools by higher education colleagues and vice versa) the temptation will be to move towards more resource-led in-service in which work is "commissioned" by schools and LEAs whose role becomes that of "purchaser". Contracts will be put out to tender and "value for money" in the limited short term economical sense of numbers and costs may become the governing factor However:

> "the real crunch comes in the relationship between these new programmes or policies and the thousands of subjective realities embedded in peoples individual and organizational contexts and their personal histories. How these subjective realities are addressed or ignored is crucial for whether potential change becomes meaningful at the level of individual use and effectiveness" (Fullan, 1982).

The course which has been described attempted to address these "subjective realities", whilst also taking direct account of institutional need. The expense involved in collaborative planning processes and the related time taken in contracting must be measured against the perceived learning of the course members and their impact upon school. "Cost effectiveness" is not simply a matter of finance but of effective learning and change.

Conclusion: De-bifurcatring research and development or writing stories together

Essentially, the kind of work described in these brief case studies is "action research". Here:

> "...all actors involved in the research process are equal participants and must be involved in every stage of the research ... It requires a special kind of communication ... which allows all participants to be partners of communication on equal terms ... collaborative participation in theorectical, practical and political discourse is thus a hallmark of action research and the action researcher ..." (Grundy and Kemmis, 1982).

In this work research and staff development are one and the same enterprise, and are both practical and emancipatory for all participants.

The model of research and professional development which underpins the work described in this chapter may be characterized as a "partnership model" in which the work does not, therefore, belong to any one individual or one interest group. It is jointly owned by each of the participants. It is an "operational relationship in which people work together towards the achievement of their goal" (Bradley, 1988), a partnership in which teachers and significant others are actively involved in negotiating processes and outcomes; and the power relationships of traditional models are avoided. The role of the external agent is to promote and sustain an environment in which discussion which provides challenge and support may occur. Erauts (1972) model of school-focused in-service education links success in helping schools solve problems to the quality of the relationship between the consultant(s) and the teacher(s). He suggests that the consultants role cannot and should not always be non-directive. The interventionist aims to seek questions which are perceived by the client as relevant to his needs, to investigate answers to these questions collaboratively and to place the onus for action on the client himself.

It is important that it is the clients voice that is heard to speak throughout the construction of the story. "Voice is a term used increasingly by researchers concerned with teacher empowerment; the term expresses an implicit critique of the prevailing tendency in earlier studies of teaching to reduce the complexity of teachers work, and to privilege theoretical formulations over the concerns of teachers themselves" (Elbaz, 1990). It is important in future years to ensure that the teachers perspective is recognised not only in the initiation of research, development and evaluation and through contracted partnerships, but also in any accounts and reports that may result. The stories (accounts, portrayals, biographies, etc.) must be written and produced in words from the particular culture of the teacher, school and society, for, "the story is not that which links teacher thought and action, for thought and action are not seen as separate domains to begin with. Rather the story is the very stuff of teaching, the landscape within which we live as teachers and researchers" (Elbaz, 1990) and within which the work of teachers and researchers can be seen as making sense. In practical terms, this means that not only must the design and processes of curriculum research and development be the result of joint planning and action, but that the written account(s) and its dissemination must reflect this. As Elbaz (1990) points out, "the fact that teacher and researcher participate in a shared discourse constitutes a small step toward the creation of a new sense of community."

Schon (1983) outlines options within professional practice, stating that:

"There are those who choose the swampy lowlands. They deliberately involve themselves in messy but crucially important problems. When asked to described their methods of inquiry, they speak of experience, trial and error, intuition, and muddling through. Other professionals opt for the high ground. Hungry for technical rigor, devoted to an image of solid technical competence, or fearful of entering a world in which they feel they do not know what they are doing, they choose to confine themselves to a narrowly technical practice ..."

It is tempting to suggest that the future for those in higher education who wish to contribute to teacher and school developments lies in choosing the lowlands. Indeed, there are those who believe that their very survival may depend on it. However, to do so they must first learn to walk in different ways, to converse in new languages and to listen to different voices. Only then will they begin to connect.

Chapter 3

PROMOTING THE ARTICULATION OF TACIT KNOWLEDGE THROUGH THE COUNSELLING OF PRACTITIONERS

Gunnar Handal, University of Oslo

Introduction: a triple pressure to work collectively

Proverbs contain condensed and confirmed truth, but they can be very conservative. One such proverb is: Speech is silver, silence is gold. The language is of course full of such expressions. Why am I so eager to break with this proverb and to see the tacit articulated; i.e. to give the practitioner voice? A reason is that silencing somebody amounts to a form of repression; while to let somebody have his say is to respect the freedom of speech. Is then, the campaign for the articulation of tacit knowledge, some sort of liberation movement for the underdog(s)? Am I championing a democratic protest with the thrust: Silent practitioners of the world, articulate!?

Joking and exaggeration aside, I think in some way practitioner research is just such a movement. And in order to make my point, I will start with a few comments on professionalization. There has been an endless discussion about whether teaching is and ought to be a profession. Most writers do not recognize it as a profession, or place it at the more obscure end of a continuum among the vocations. Teaching possesses few of the characteristics required to be recognized as a profession according to the sociological criteria: the scientific knowledge-base is questionable, experienced teachers have little autonomy to sanction novices, there is no own code of ethics, et cetera. In consequence the teaching vocation's dream of becoming professional, is probably in vain.

But there is a different form of professionalism which can be defined as the opposite of being an amateur. The amateur is someone who practices within a field without having been properly taught; who does something for fun or in order to save the costs of having it done by a real master of the trade. We all do this, when we paint our house, fix our car, or try to cut the hair of our children.

The first type of professionalism is a quality accredited to a vocation by society; accordingly it is a societal and historic phenomenon that can change over time and place. The latter, the non-amateurish professionalism, exists in all vocations with a sufficient body of expertise; it is what distinguishes someone who is really good at something from the sufficient or mediocre.

My point is that teaching is an undertaking that is so complex and requires such a high degree of competence to be carried out professionally, that really good teaching, professionally done, is not a job for amateurs. The problem is that given the size and cost of education in modern society, its societal tradition and the importance really acknowledged to education (when all exaggerations of rhetoric have been left aside), it is generally assumed that the job can be mastered by someone who falls short of genuine professional status.

I am not an eager soldier in the battle to achieve social recognition for teaching as a profession. In my eyes this struggle is often aimed at trying to live up to the formal criteria of professionalism: giving basic teacher education programmes a more "scientific" content, establishing rules that inhibit "unauthorized" persons from working in schools or setting up committees to develop a common code of ethics. As an educationalist and not a teacher union leader, I am more concerned with establishing the other professionalism; to see to it that teaching is not a profession inhabited by amateurs. The risk of this strategy is that the occupation might earn being classified as a profession and not have this societally recognized. Central to this other professionalism is one's concern with the quality of teacher work. Of course the criteria we establish and the demands we make on quality teaching, are societally, culturally and historically defined. Therefore the discussion of the other professionalism has to be grounded in a consideration of a specific situation; I choose the one I know the best, that of the Norwegian school system.

Generally the work of teachers is described as dominated by individualism. This fact is rather well established and documented in research. The teacher's role has been portrayed, in terms of collegiality, as a lonely one. Teachers supposedly lack a common "technical culture" (Lortie, 1975), are weak in "teaching expertise" and are little willing to take on a "professional role". (Buchmann, 1984)

I see in my own country, however, clear signs of an increasing emphasis on teaching as a collective task. This has particularly to do with a change in the character of the Norwegian national curriculum. Norway has a long tradition of having a common national curriculum, particularly on the elementary school level, but even at the secondary one. This curriculum used to be quite specific, particularly concerning content; but also on issues of method. The teacher was cast in the role of an implementer of set plans. An even older tradition – though still alive – saw the teacher as a charismatic cultural agent exerting his/her educative influence on new generations, fairly independently of any curricular directions. The curriculum, when construed as a rather detailed prescription for teachers' work, provided a framework where the individual teacher with reasonable success could carry out his/her work under the model of "my classroom is my castle". The process of executing set plans according to specified rules could be reasonably well mastered individually.

Recent developments in Norway have produced a different type of national curriculum. It is referred to as a "frame curriculum", which implies that the decisions are left to the teachers concerning what to teach (within broadly defined subject areas), when to teach it, and how to teach it. The traditional school subjects still exist – more or less – as do rather precise allocations of time. But within the subjects, curriculum content is merely defined in broad areas with examples given of topics and themes which are to be considered as mere suggestions. This type of curriculum could be described metaphorically as a menu where the dishes can be selected according to taste, where you have to help yourself to entrée, soup, main course and desert; and where you may not reduce the menu to only one course.

This situation has existed for approximately fifteen years. The last curriculum reform in 1987, made this curriculum concept all the more pronounced. Until then the majority of teachers did not seem to fully understand the intentions of the concept. Thus it was considered necessary to impose additional demands on the schools in order to make practice change. Now schools are required to establish local versions of the national curriculum for their own school, indicating what they will focus on and how they are going to teach in order to fulfill the national requirements. And to top it all off, schools have been required to develop plans for locally based school improvement, in accordance with their local curriculum and in order to gradually approach the ideals expressed in it.

Motivated by the same ideological tenets as the local curriculum, pressure has been applied through the frame curriculum as well as through in-service courses in favor of team teaching. A redefinition of teachers' work in the direction of more collective practice has resulted. It is no longer sufficient for the local school, in order to fulfill its obligations, to guarantee the quality of individual teacher's work. Many of the tasks now expected of the school can hardly be dealt with properly without collective teacher action.

The 1987 curriculum reform for grades 1 to 9 adopted a decentralized school-based improvement strategy. The development and implementation at each and every school, of a local version of the national frame curriculum was intended as an element of this strategy. The drafting of this local version of the curriculum is supposed to be a collective effort, undertaken by the teachers in each school. Thus an important collective task has been introduced in a working environment where previously the job could be mastered reasonably well through pure individual effort.

A reform in the working hours of teachers has accompanied the initiatives already described. Until 1989 Norwegian teachers were only required to be on the school premises for the lessons they taught. Apart from this, they were free to work at home or anywhere else. The reform has introduced a new requirement; teachers must work at least five hours a week on the school premises in addition to the lessons they teach. This is considered to be, more or less, collective time wherein cooperative work involving one's colleagues is supposed to take place. The teachers' unions have not accepted this new arrangement without a fight, although the attitudes among the teachers themselves were quite mixed. At many primary and lower secondary schools similar arrangements had in fact previously been established on a voluntary basis.

Thus a triple pressure on schools and teachers to work more collectively has been formed by:
- the establishment of collective tasks,
- the provision of collective time to solve them, and
- the ideological pressure on teachers to work together.

What has happened under such a circumstance? In order to answer this question I need to clarify some concepts which I can then use to provide an answer.

Levels of practice

It has been well documented that personal practical theories of work underlay the practice of teaching, although this phenomenon has been given various names by the different researchers (Polanyi, 1958; Elbaz, 1983; Connelly & Clandinin, 1985; Clark & Peterson, 1986; Handal & Lauvås, 1987). Such personal practical theories of work consist to a large extent of tacit / implicit knowledge and competences. This knowledge exists over and beyond that which the holder can readily formulate. This non-formulated level has intra-subjective meaning; it exists inside the subject and affects his/her practice but it is not communicated verbally to others. Such knowledge is acquired via practical work, often in direct contact with competent actors and in situations where the knowledge is used. In the reservoir of tacit knowledge there may also be knowledge, skills and attitudes acquired a long time ago in the formulated form, which have become part of the tacit, taken for granted level, and which it is no longer found necessary to formulate.

Although some tacit knowledge or competence probably never can or should be formulated, much individual teacher tacit knowledge can be formulated, even if at a particular moment it has not already occurred.

So far we have been dealing with the individual level; a similar concept is to be identified on the collective level i.e. of the school or the group of teachers. Arfwedson (1985) uses the concept of school codes or collective codes to discuss the tacit knowledge of groups of teachers. In his terminology a school code of a particular school "consists of an 'aggregate' of guiding principles for interpretation and action, embracing whatever is important with reference to work, work environment and problems in this school." (Arfwedson, 1985, p. 31) These guiding principles help teachers in a particular school to organize the world around them in a meaningful and consistent way. Thus the school code, as defined by Arfwedson, comes very close to the idea of a collective practical theory of work for teachers within the same school. Although there may be differences between individual teacher codes within a staff, or there may be conflicting codes held by groups of teachers within the same school (as Arfwedson also found in his empirical research), there is still a common school code regulating the interpretations and practices of the collective of teachers. You will not find the school code framed and hanging on the wall of the staff room. As with individual practical theories of teaching, the school code is largely taken for granted; practitioners find it neither necessary to formulate nor to substantiate their school code. The school code contains a number of underlying assumptions (Schein, 1983) which implicitly and uncritically influence interpretations made and actions taken within the school. As these assumptions are not formulated, they escape reflection and critical examination. Consequently there is a risk that the code will have a conservative effect on practice. Only through communication will intra-subjective, personal theories of practice become intersubjectively available, and can actors holding different practical theories examine and confront one another's positions. Such a confrontation may influence the collective theory of the school – the school code – because implicit assumptions of practice will become available for collective discussion.

When teaching becomes more collective, as has occurred in Norway, through work on the local curriculum, it will not be sufficient to make suggestions on the basis of an implicit personal practical theory of teaching. Teachers will have to be able to express the reasons for accepting these suggestions. This will require three things:
- the formulation and development of teacher's personal practical theories.
- the development of skills for dealing with these, partly different, individual practical theories; in order to integrate them and to base curricular decisions and practice on them.
- a forum and time for the afore mentioned.

This is partly a question of individual competence, partly one of collective competence; and partly one of favorable circumstances..

Firstly to examine the individual aspect: in our own work (Handal & Lauvås, 1987) we have (based on Lövlie, 1974) distinguished three levels in the concept of practice:

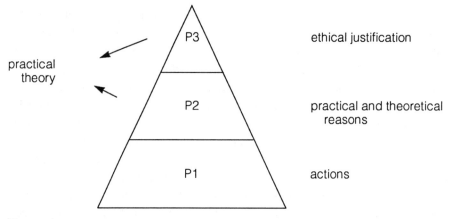

Figure 1

Teachers identify the concept of practice with the P1 level of action, while all three levels can be validly included in the concept. The reasons (at level P2) why we act as we do (at level P1) are an important part of our actions which give them meaning and sense; as are the ethical (and political) justifications (level P3) that we use to defend morally why we find it acceptable to act in a particular way. At the P2 and P3 levels we make use of knowledge (theoretical and experiential, tacit and formulated) and values which form our personal practical theories of teaching. An integrated concept of practice, such as I am presenting here, includes both practical theory as well as actions.

In the strategy for counselling or tutoring teachers that we have developed, the focus is on the articulation and development of the teacher's practical theory of teaching (Handal & Lauvås, 1987). The counselling takes place in pre- and post-teaching sessions, on the basis of a written "counselling document" formulated by the teacher in response to a practical teaching situation (widely defined). The focus of the counselling is not on polishing the teacher's performance. Rather the primary focus is on reflecting on the knowledge and values underlying the planning and implementation of teaching. The actual teaching session is used in an exemplaric way, where the counselling focuses on those aspects of the situation which provide grounds for discussing more general issues related to teaching. The discussion aims at all three levels of the triangle of practice described above, and thus serves to make conscious and articulate elements of the personal practical theory of the teacher.

We have experiential evidence that such reflective counselling over time increases the teachers' awareness of the reasons why behind their actual teaching. The tutor's role in this process is: partly to elicit explanations, reasons and justifications in an honestly interested and non-judging way; and partly to look seriously and critically into the reasons given, possibly in order to confront them with alternative knowledge, experience and values.

To be successful the process of counselling (tutoring) has to be carried out according to several central principles. One of them has been mentioned above: the principle of the exemplaric approach to the practice [teaching] discussed. In addition, there are three principles:

- During the counselling the dialogue between the teacher and the counsellor/ tutor is focused on a situation and specific context. The teacher's practical theory is not discussed in decontextualized abstraction, but in close relationship to actual teaching events. This limits the idealistic (and often ideological) nature of discussion and the arguments used. What can be learned in such a discussion therefore influences more readily the teacher's practical theory. No one can, by definition, formulate their personal, practical [tacit] theory of teaching when asked to do so. In trying, we end up with very general and abstract statements which seem to have limited influence on practical theories.

- The quality of the dialogue during counselling is of great importance. Serious conversation about teaching is often referred to as discussion, and carries with it connotations of debate. This includes a tacit expectation that somebody will win (most often the tutor) and the other party will loose (most often the teacher). This does not create a productive climate for learning. An alternative is the socially amiable dialogue where everybody states their opinion, nobody gets hurt and where not much is learned.

Counselling should, as an ideal, have the qualities of a discourse: a power free dialogue between equal partners seeking understanding together of a topic or a problem of mutual interest, where the better argument is respected. The persons engaged in the counselling discourse are jointly engaged in understanding the teaching being considered. No one of them has the power to define the situation or to authorize any right answers. No one is forced to choose between accepting, submitting or rebelling. These criteria may not be satisfied very often in normal counselling, but I am convinced that they still should be affirmed as an ideal to strive for. The ideal makes a world of a difference in the concrete results of the counselling.

- The third principle also relates to the nature of the communication in counselling. There are many tacit expectations in a counselling relationship that need to be brought out into the open, particularly if the counsellor tries to practice a strategy of counselling such as reflective counselling which is unknown to his/her target group. The underlying reasons why have to be clarified if teachers are to feel themselves comfortable. Otherwise the counsellor may be trying to follow a trail for which the teacher has no map. Such situations in counselling call for metacommunication in the widest sense of the word: communication about communication, communication about the relationship between the persons concerned, communication about the counselling strategy. This metacommunication is not restricted to an introductory period characterized by the clarification of terms; it is most fruitfully used on and off throughout the counselling discourse. We have even found it helpful, to use "time" out the same way as it is used in basketball; as a physical sign for an interruption of the topic led discourse in order to make explicative or questioning comments on communication and process.

Hunting for collective reflection in the school

To return to the question posed previously: what happens when the school and its teachers have been confronted with new collective tasks; time has been provided to deal with these tasks; and pressure has been put on the teachers to cooperate in their work? It sounds like an ideal situation for the school to develop into a more collective work community.

I found myself, during the academic year 1989-90, in the final phase of a research project in just this context. That academic year I followed with two colleagues three schools which were implementing the reform calling for teachers to spend five hours per week in addition to their actual classroom teaching, in the school. One of the schools was a rural elementary school (grade 1 to 6) with fifteen teachers; another was an urban lower secondary school (grade 7 to 9) with approximately thirty teachers, and the last school was an urban upper secondary comprehensive school (grade 10 to 12) with approximately forty teachers. I will focus on the elementary school, called here Woodland, which best illustrates my points. At Woodland the staff had mixed feelings about the reform, due mostly to differences in their private situations (full versus part time jobs, married or not, with/without small children, etc). A limited version of the reform had been tried out the previous year. Small groups of colleagues had tried to assist or counsel each other in their work. The new situation with five extra hours per week in school was, however, a significant change which was welcomed by some but not by others.

The five hours of collective time was organized as follows: two hours were scheduled Monday after school to qualify the teachers for Cooperative learning and Process writing. These themes had been included in the local school development plan. Two pairs of teachers had taken in-service courses in these methods, to be able to train their colleagues. Two times a week an hour was set aside before the children came to school. One morning was used for a short meeting to keep staff informed of current matters and to expedite routine decision making not requiring lengthy discussion. More fundamental, complex or controversial decisions were left for staff meetings held an evening every second month. The other morning was reserved for consultation of the teacher teams working in the same or parallel classes; these teams also had an hour scheduled as a part of their normal teaching load. One hour per week was left open for each teacher to deal individually with matters which needed to take place at school such as talking to pupils and/or parents; parent-teacher meetings, et cetera. Most of the additional in-school time was reserved for collective work, either in a plenary or small group format. The intentions of the reform were respected.

Three observations on teacher use of collective time from my research can be presented:

1. The Monday afternoon two hour sessions were, I believe, a very constructive element in staff development. Alternating between two topics (Cooperative Learning and Process Writing) the teachers who had followed the in-service courses taught their colleagues the ideas and methods they had acquired. Theoretical presentations were combined with practical exercises. Suggestions and discussion of classroom implementation for differing subjects, levels and grades, followed. Tasks were formulated to try out during the week; from time to time (twice a semester) report sessions were organized to describe what had been tried out, how it had worked and what commentary there was. The teachers arranged between one another to observer each other's classes, when new practice was being tried out. Some made video recordings which were later shown and discussed. Advice for further practice was then formulated. This was, thus, an instance of school based improvement; planned and implemented by colleagues who taught and counselled each other, in the context of a school improvement project. All this was experienced very positively by the entire staff. A collective attitude was created where it was common to talk about and to share personal teaching experiences both of a negative and a positive kind. Teacher pride in what they were doing grew, as did external recognition for their achievements. Furthermore, this happened at a school which had not been a model of collective work, which was not considered progressive or particularly professional, but which did have a generally friendly atmosphere and a low level of conflict.

2. What also struck me was an observation on another level, which not only applied to the project just described, but to the whole spectrum of intercollegial cooperation. Teacher cooperation was directed to a very large extent to planning; teachers talked about What to do, When to do it, How to do it and Who should do what. To put it more generally: they engaged in preparation and implementation. In my terms they were planning at the level of action or P1. Very rarely did they refer to any reasons (P2) or justifications for (P3) the actions being planned. This could be due to the fact that between people who work closely together, as cooperating teachers do, it is not constantly necessary to formulate the reasons behind actions. One could assume that the reasons have been stated in past discussions and do not need to be repeated or reformulated

over and over again. All those involved know them anyway. But when I asked the teachers to formulate their reasons and justifications for my benefit, they experienced that it was difficult for them to do so. We are not used to do that, they said, and when you ask us to do so, we realize that we don't really have clear reasons why we plan to teach in this particular way. After several such experiences, some of the teachers became aware of their lack of P2 and P3 reasoning in relation to the actual planning of their practice. Their spontaneous comment on this theme during planning situations was: Don't ask! We know that we cannot state the reasons why we decide to do it this way, but we know it works.

There was nothing particularly complicated or unusual about the teaching they were planning. It was certainly adequate; some of it was really very good, some less distinguished. The teachers were neither particularly well qualified, nor weak. There was, however, in their cooperative work a systematic concentration on the action level. Though one might expect that there would be at least some need to communicate individual or common practical theories of action, this did not take place. When explicitly asked to formulate themselves on the level of their underlying theories, the teachers were not particularly successful in doing so; further they reported that this was for them an unusual activity. The teachers tended to focus on the procedures, methods and possible contents of teaching. New methods were quickly integrated in individual and collective preparation, as well as implementation, of teaching. But even when relatively new demands were made, there were only rare references to questions of why.

I want to stress that there is no moral judgment in what I am saying. The examples given are not instances of teacher malpractice. In fact, the same phenomenon was found in the other two schools we researched. In my view we are dealing with a generally occurring phenomenon. Within the school as institution, the actors are subject to the coercion to act. In their work, a large percentage of time is in situations where they have to act on the spot. Teachers have to attend continuously to a changing classroom situation which makes it impossible to do exactly what one has prepared. Furthermore, the classroom leaves one little chance for reflection. This type of activity fills a lot of the day. When there is time for preparation it seems more practical to look forward to the coming day and to focus on what to do then, than to look back and evaluate past actions or to reflect in general, on one's plans of action. Furthermore, teachers' theories of practice are to a large extent tacit and are comprised of experiences and values acquired in action and mostly taken for granted. Unless the teacher is further qualified and motivated for such an activity, his/her ideas are easily left unformulated. In addition, reasons and justifications at the P2 and P3 levels are often not in demand in teacher culture. Cooperating teachers share a lot of common, taken for granted and tacit knowledge. P2 and P3 questioning could upset all that.

3. During the time I spent at Woodland School, it was discovered that I had worked extensively in the counselling of teachers. I was immediately requested to run a one day workshop for staff on inter-colleague counselling. As a researcher, I was in a dilemma. On the one hand it was only fair that I made a contribution to the school, in response to all the help they'd given me in my research. On the other, I might interfere in the natural course of school development by introducing a set of concepts and practices that otherwise would not have been known. The evident social justice of the request predominated over the reservations of the researcher (which were not very strong anyway, as my work much more resembled an ethnographic study than a controlled experiment).

I spent a day with the staff talking about personal and collective practical theories of teaching, going through simple exercises of collegial counselling, and focusing on the need for formulation and discourse on the P2 and P3 levels. I also joined the staff on a two day staff development seminar later in the year. At that time they were more strongly interested in applying a P2/P3 perspective on their own teaching practice, but still not very able to do so.

The following example is illustrative: the programme included a demonstration of an example of teaching, which used a combination of process writing and cooperative learning; that was followed by discussion mainly on the P1 level. When I asked: Why they would like to teach this way, What it might mean to different groups of pupils, How they would handle different reactions from parents, and Why they would do so, they regarded these as very pertinent and relevant questions and discussed them at some length. However this type of discourse did not occur spontaneously between them. The reaction from some of the staff towards the end of the discussion was that the group needed to talk through their concepts of knowledge and learning, their views and values related to pupils and parents. The need for such clarification is probably correct. However a general, abstract, decontextualized discussion will probably generate less clarification than an exemplaric discourse related to an example at hand. The way of stating their need, indicates the fundamental split inherent in much of our thinking between theory or philosophy on the one hand (as separate domains of study) and practice on the other (with its emphasis on unreflected action).

Teachers, in order to fulfill their role in transforming a frame (of reference) curriculum into daily practice through a process of school improvement, need to develop their qualifications for collective reflection on work. This is a qualification which the typical school staff does not possess; the nature and tradition of the job coerces teachers into concentrating on the action aspect of work. Carr and Kemmis (1986) refer to this development process as action research:

"Action research aims at improvement in three areas: firstly the improvement of a practice; secondly, the improvement of the understanding of the practice by its practitioners; and thirdly, the improvement of the situation in which the practice takes place. ... It can be argued that these three conditions are individually necessary and jointly sufficient for action research to be said to exist: firstly, a project takes as its subject matter a social practice regarding it as a form of strategic action susceptible of improvement; secondly, the project proceeds through a spiral of cycles of planning, acting, observing and reflecting, ...thirdly, the project involves those responsible for the practice in each of the moments of the activity ..." (p. 165)

They clarify this further through the following figure: (p. 186)

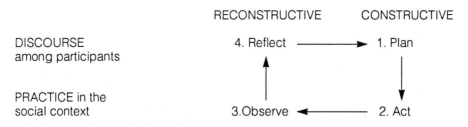

Figure 2

My own research shows that the bulk of activity in cooperative work among teachers is constructive and very little is reconstructive. An explanation for this is sought in the coercion to act inherent in the classroom situation and in the culture of teaching. The normal situation in a school-based school-improvement process seems to be that of an incomplete self-reflective spiral. The consequence is some improvement of practice (or rather of action), but little improvement in understanding nor in the situation where the action takes place. Structural awareness or contextual analysis just does not get off the ground. There may be change, but far less systematic and fundamental improvement takes place than Carr and Kemmis foresee. At Woodland action changed in fundamentally good ways, but the attitude of "treating what counts as knowledge as problematic" (Carr and Kemmis, p. 85) or of studying critically one's own practice, was not yet achieved. Change was mainly on the P1 level of action.

In conclusion two questions

1. Is it important to champion a critical, self reflective attitude as a necessary norm for teachers and schools?
2. Can such a norm be realized?

I think it is essential that teachers in schools form self-critical, self-reflecting communities. My main reason for this lies in the type of job teachers are contracted to take on. The education of future generations of persons in a quickly changing pluralistic society, cannot be adequately undertaken in a technical way according to pre-defined rules and regulations by actors who have little personal or collective understanding of their job. It is not sufficient to have good craftsmen or bureaucrats. We need professionals (in the sense of the word defined above). If we go for less, the result will probably be a group of dissatisfied and frustrated teachers jumping from one bandwagon to another; or teachers who keep both feet so firmly on the ground that they cannot move at all. This picture has few similarities with that sketched by the action-researchers of the systematic improvement of schools. Although we may see elements of the negative pictures in today's schools, it is not an accurate appraisal of the general situation. There is definitely significant movement going on out there.

Consequently my answer to the second question is also: yes. It can be done, although this answer is a bit more reluctantly pronounced. I feel confident that we are on the right track when teachers accept to solve collective tasks, and are thus confronted with a demand for discourse in order to prove themselves able to make decisions at the curricular level. It is necessary that time is provided for the carrying out of collective critical self-reflection. Probably teachers have far less time and opportunity to work collectively than is necessary. In my view there is a pressing need in a large proportion of schools to provide stimulus and assistance in developing competence for this type of professional work. The potential is there; the frames for developing it are partly established; the competence is still to a large extent lacking.

This is where counselling, tutoring, facilitation, guidance or whatever we will call it, comes in. It is a difficult, challenging, and from time to time threatening activity; to look at oneself, one's colleagues and the job we are doing together in a critical way; knowing you risk to find it professionally unsatisfactory and knowing you will then have to do something about it to improve it. A climate, and particularly a competence, is needed for this to be possible. In most cases intervention will be needed from outside, in the form of a critical friend; not in the form of a controller or a missionary for a particular cause. Carr and Kemmis (1986) put it this way:

"... outsiders can legitimately take a kind of facilitatory role in establishing self-reflective communities of action researchers. ... the 'moderator' can help to form a self-critical and self-reflective community, but, once it has formed, it is the responsibility of the community itself to sustain and develop its work. Any continuing dominance of a 'moderator' will be destructive of the collaborative responsibility of the group for its own self-reflection." (p. 205)

This way of thinking outlines a role for facilitation or counselling, where the focus is on assisting teachers in discovering: a common language; ways in which they can describe, observe and reflect upon their practice; and strategies for establishing this way of working as a central part to their job. In other words a type of meta-language and meta-knowledge is being proposed which makes it possible to approach the practice of teaching critically. This meta-language is at present only occasionally present within the vocation. It must be developed in close relationship to work carried out in schools. What goes on in planning and teaching, preparation and evaluation, and all other sorts of day-to-day practice has to be articulated. It is easy to confound this sort of qualification on the meta-level, with qualifications for (for instance) particular ways of teaching. Nevertheless we are dealing with different types of qualifications: one for teaching and the other for talking and thinking about teaching as well as for reflecting on teaching practice.

In order to develop the necessary meta-competence, teachers must formulate their tacit knowledge, share it with colleagues and gradually establish a collective understanding of practice. At the same time teachers must develop the meta-language and meta-knowledge to change debates into discourses and action into praxis. If we can make this happen, there will no longer be any doubt about the professionalism of teachers. Consequently, and returning to my starting point, I also see this process as one of the liberation or emancipation of the teaching vocation.

❖❖ II ❖❖

VARIOUS APPROACHES TO THE PROFESSIONAL DEVELOPMENT OF TEACHERS AND SCHOOLS

THE PROVISION OF PROFESSIONAL DEVELOPMENT FOR TEACHERS

Les Bell, University of Warwick

My theme is the professional development of teachers. My title may lead you to expect that I am going to explore what happens when teachers make their own choices about the form that such development should take and, to some extent, this will be addressed. Of greater significance, however, is the framework within which such choices are made and the inter-relationship between the patterning of choices and the nature of the provision that is made for teachers' professional development. In order to deal in depth with this inter-relationship I shall begin by examining briefly the most pervasive form of professional development. In the second section I shall then discuss three different but overlapping models of professional development provision, exploring some of the tensions within each of them and highlighting the extent to which development needs to occur on three organisational levels within schools. The final section will consider some of the implications for schools, teachers, local education authorities and institutions of higher education of the choices that have to be made about the professional development of teachers.

The professional development of teachers: apprenticeship or process?

My first experience of any form of professional development as a teacher took place in the early 1960s during my probationary year. I was given a classroom across the corridor from a dynamic and creative deputy headteacher in a primary school in Penge. I was so impressed by the impact of his visual display and his ability to stimulate a group of tough, cynical youngsters that I welcomed the opportunity to team-teach with him. We conducted a survey of local beauty spots which involved taking 80 children to a wooded area in a large red bus. The work was planned in detail and the children, in mixed age and ability groups, were given specific tasks to complete on identified parts of the area in a limited time. The work was duly carried out as planned. We did not lose or gain a single child. We caused no disturbance to any flora or fauna except for an unfortunate and embarrassing encounter with an early morning courting couple. Those city children came to realise how fascinating such a study could be. Their subsequent work formed the basis for a mobile display that won prizes at the local county show. I acquired skills of planning, organisation and creating displays by working with my more experienced colleague. I felt that my development as a professional teacher had really started. This all happened entirely by accident as, I suspect, did much of the professional development of most teachers at that time. I did, however, choose to become involved in the team teaching process.

Much of the rest of my development as a teacher took place in the same random, almost haphazard way through chance encounters with colleagues. My experience was typical of that of my peers. We tended to learn about our professional roles and to acquire the related skills by working alongside other teachers. This apprenticeship model of career development is characteristic of most occupations. However, for teachers it also builds on their experience as students. Indeed the sociological concept of 'anticipatory socialisation' sums up the way in which prospective entrants into an occupation consciously and unconsciously study the characteristics of the people already in a job and take on the attitudes, values, behaviour patterns and even appearance of members of that occupation. Many professional habits – good and bad – emerge during this process. Much of what we learned as teachers came from our day-to-day contact with colleagues, but this is a limited and insufficient form of development. For example:

a. The role models which are available may not be good role models for an inexperienced teacher to follow.
b. The team of teachers encountered may not be particularly united or effective.
c. The experience that a particular member of staff may need in order to update his or her skills or knowledge may not be present in the school or place involved.
d. A passive approach to staff development by which staff learn solely by association with colleagues is not consistent with the need to manage schools and develop them in a coherent, planned and structured way.

It is also arguable how far such experiences are truly developmental. They may help an individual teacher to acquire skills but such an activity would only be developmental if it enabled the teachers to make a planned contribution to the work of the school based on:

a. a self-analysis of professional needs and effectiveness;
b. an analysis of the needs and effectiveness of the school;
c. identifying and achieving a set of goals related to both levels of analysis.

My random apprenticeship met none of these criteria. Nor did it fit easily into the categories of "further professional study" or "staff development" that Taylor (1975) identified. He defined "further professional study" as being "orientated to the needs of individual teachers" while staff development was "rooted in the needs of the institution". (Taylor, 1975, pp 5-6) A year later, however, we find Watson arguing that, "The term staff development refers to the activity of ensuring the personal and professional development of the staff of the school." (Watson, 1976, p 18) This definition implies the need to devise processes for professional development which will attempt to secure the professional growth of the teacher, whilst, at the same time, improving the performance of both teachers and schools.

The reasoning behind the general support given to professional development in educational organisations rests on the assumption that the interdependent relationship of the school and the teacher is crucial: a teacher cannot improve his or her performance consistently if the organisation is in poor health, and the total functioning of the school rests on the sum of the individual teachers' contribution. Therefore, if the organisation can harmonise the individuals' wishes for personal and career development with the requirements of the organisation as derived from its educational aims, it will improve individual and organisational performance. The teacher, the school and the pupils should benefit from such a process. Professional development in these terms implies the involvement of the whole staff in the operation and management of the school. It also implies that much of the work of staff development must be directed towards the improvement of the school as well as the professional advancement of individuals. Professional development thus has three major strands and takes place at three different organisational levels:

a. the personal development of individual teachers through the acquisition of skills and competencies;
b. the development of groups of teachers working as teams, departments or units;
c. the planned corporate development of the whole school.

However, there are potential tensions between these different levels of staff development. Staff at various stages in their careers, and with different interests and personal circumstances, have contrasting needs and ideas about their work and how it might develop. These may differ from the needs and ideas of their colleagues. Different groups within the school might find themselves competing for the same scarce resources, while the needs of individuals and groups might be at odds with those of the whole school. How can these areas of potential conflict be reconciled and what are the implications of enabling the teachers within the schools to make choices about staff development? In order to address these issues it is necessary to look at the ways in which the strategies adopted by teachers to achieve professional development have changed in recent years.

Approaches to the professional development of teachers

We can now see that the professional development of teachers should, in an ideal world, be regarded as:

"a deliberate and continuous process involving the identification and discussion of present and anticipated needs of individual staff for furthering their job satisfaction and career prospects and of the institution for supporting its academic work and plans, and the implementation of programmes of staff activities designed for the harmonious satisfaction of needs." (Billings, 1977, p 22)

Thus the process of development caters both for the individual needs of teachers and for the policy needs of the whole school as well as those of its constituent parts. I use the term professional development to encompass all such developmental activities within schools, since my main intention is to explore the choices that are made about professional development by all those involved and to examine some of the implications of those choices.

Such a view cannot conceal the conflicts that are inherent in any programme of professional development. Individual teachers will want a process that caters for their personal self-improvement and which acknowledges the difficulties and complexities of the job. On the other hand, heads and senior staff will want a form of development that reflects their assessment of the needs of the school and the demands on it which emanate from parents, governors and other stakeholders. At the same time the Local Education Authority (LEA) will want to ensure that its priorities are given prominence while the Ministry of Education sets and resources its own national priorities for the development of teachers. These different perceptions influence the nature of the support that has been provided for teachers. They help to create a framework within which practitioner choices about professional development are made.

Apart from the apprenticeship model of professional development, if the term can be applied to such a random and haphazard series of largely unconnected activities, it is possible to identify three main types of professional development provision that have been available to teachers. These are:

1. development through in-service education and training (INSET) courses;
2. development through school-focused and school-based programmes;
3. development through whole-school policy implementation.

Each approach both requires and enables teachers, acting collectively or as individuals, to make a series of choices about their professional development. Each approach contains its own set of assumptions about the nature and purposes of professional development and how best to facilitate that development within schools. These three approaches have always existed. At the margins, the boundaries between them are extremely blurred. As models of professional development provision, however, they enable us to identify some of the key issues associated with the process of providing professional support for teachers. I will examine each of the models in turn, showing its main features, assumptions and weaknesses and identifying how these are related to the subsequent form of provision. The models are summarised in table 1.

Professional development through courses

The course-based model of professional development was, and still is, the most common and widely accepted approach to the development of teachers. For many, professional development is "going on a course." As Henderson (1979) has shown, the notion of taking teachers out of school and instructing them in groups had its origins in the nineteenth century. Its rationale lay in the need to improve the education of relatively poorly educated teachers and, as such, it was probably highly effective. In more recent times, however, the treatment of newly qualified teachers was based on the assumption that initial training provided teachers with all the expertise that they required for the rest of their professional life.

In-service courses tended, therefore, to fall into three groups. The first was for the enhancement of existing qualifications so that non-graduates could become graduates and those with degrees could obtain higher degrees or diplomas. These courses tended to be theoretical, based in institutions of higher education and were grounded in what the staff of those institutions could and would provide rather than on any considered analysis of the needs of teachers and their schools. Here it was assumed that improved qualifications would in some way enhance professional performance. Until recently, the provision of such long, full-time award bearing courses for teachers on secondment provided a major source of employment for staff in education departments in institutions of higher education. The second and third types of courses are closely related and often indistinguishable. They are the top-up and the remedial courses. The top-up courses are intended to further develop existing professional skills. The remedial courses help teachers in areas in which they are perceived to be experiencing difficulty. The current rash of primary school science courses generated by the demands of the national curriculum provides an example. Often these courses are run by local authority advisers, sometimes working with teachers but universities and colleges are also significant providers along with a range of other agencies.

The provision of courses grew rapidly in the 1970s and course attendance by teachers increased dramatically (Henderson, 1979). Professional development through attending courses became a panacea for improving the quality of schools and the education of children. In spite of this there was little evaluation of the impact of courses on the work of teachers in schools. The intention was that the teacher returning from the course would be able to identify those elements of the course work that were relevant to his or her classroom practice and that he or she would then be able to apply such expertise in the context of his or her day-to-day work. This, in turn, would then have an effect on colleagues within the school. They would recognise the virtues of the good practice being demonstrated by the new, improved, course stimulated teacher and would seek to emulate what they observed.

This approach to professional development assumes that change in schools can be brought about by changing selected or even randomly self-selected individuals within those schools. They will then successfully generate change in others to such an extent that the school itself will be transformed. This is what Georgiades and Phillimore have termed:

> "... the myth of the hero-innovator: the idea that you can produce, by training, a knight in shining armour who, loins girded with new technology and beliefs, will assault his organisational fortress and institute changes both in himself and others at stroke. Such a view is ingenuous. The fact of the matter is that organisations such as schools will, like dragons, eat hero innovators for breakfast." (Georgiades and Phillimore, 1975, p 134)

This was not the only limitation of professional development through INSET courses. Courses of this type tend to emphasise the expertise of those outside schools and to deny the legitimacy of the teacher-as-expert. This is an almost inevitable result of organising the provision of staff development in this way. It tended to perpetuate the demand for courses in spite of there often being a mismatch between the needs of teachers and/or their schools and the content of the courses. At the same time the provision of courses was unsystematic and unplanned, reflecting the existence of a plethora of providing agencies; the need on the part of these agencies to offer what expertise they had to provide rather than to offer what teachers and schools needed and wanted; and the failure to establish appropriate feedback and follow-up mechanisms for such courses even when provided within and by LEAs.

Nevertheless, courses remain a popular form of professional development for teachers. They do enable teachers to make choices. The most obvious choice that teachers can make is whether or not to become involved. Those who so choose can decide to enhance their qualifications, to develop existing skills or to acquire new skills. They can also choose when and where to undertake such courses. They are offered the possibility of secondment, although this is now unlikely to be available to the majority of teachers. Teachers can also make choices about what, if anything, they choose to apply and how they choose to apply it. They may wish to practice new skills within the security of their own classroom. They may wish to work with other members of their team or department. They may wish to share with the whole school some of their expertise or they may choose to do nothing at all.

Teachers are aware of the limitations of this form of professional development for reasons which will be explored in the next two sub-sections. As a result they are now making more informed choices about course selection. These choices tend to operate at two levels. The first relates to the course itself. Increasingly, teachers selecting courses are looking for detailed information about courses including: precise information details about who the course has been designed for in terms of job, scope of responsibility, experience; course objectives stated in terms of what course members will be able to do as a result of attending the course; course content including subject matter, specific skills and timing; the range of teaching techniques to be used and facilities to be provided; size of the group and information about course tutors and the providing agency; the provision of course evaluation and post-course follow-up; the duration, venue and cost of the course.

Teachers are thus seeking to make more informed choices about courses and to relate course choice to planned professional development. At the same time, more effort is being made to ensure that colleagues within schools benefit from the experience gained by the teacher attending the course. The impetus for this comes, from the fact that attendance at courses may now be funded from the school's own budget. Even where this is not the case, attendance may have to be justified in terms of the overall development plan for the school. As a result teachers may be: briefed before attending courses about what they may be expected to do as a result of attending the course; produce an action plan as a result of attending the course; make arrangements for applying new skills in their classroom or within the schools; expected to provide in-service training within the school, based on their own expertise; asked to provide an evaluation of the course in terms of its value to them and to their school.

Increasingly, attempts are made to ensure that courses are relevant to the needs of teachers and their schools. The focus is increasing on how far those teachers who attend courses can make a more professional contribution to the effectiveness of their institution and can improve the quality of education provided pupils. As a result, the ownership of courses, their content, methodology and evaluation, is shifting away from the providers and towards the consumers. No longer are courses planned by providers alone. Teachers are being involved in planning and identifying appropriate topics. The choices that practitioners make are determining the nature of the course provision in a very real way. Nevertheless, many of the weaknesses in this model of professional development provision still remain.

School-based and school-focused programs of professioal development

There are thus major problems surrounding the traditional course-based approach to professional development. External courses may be too theoretical and not sufficiently related to classroom practice; such courses may have little reference to school needs; simplistic assumptions may be made about the ways in which schools change and can be changed; and the role played by those outside schools in determining the structure and content of such courses may be counter-productive. These concerns led a number of different groups who were interested in the quality of in-service provision available to teachers to search for alternative strategies for professional development. These strategies tended to fall into one of two categories, the school-based or the school-focused approaches.

The school-based model was based on the view that the school, acting as a learning community,

> "could identify and solve many of its problems including the INSET needs of its staff. The school would, if sufficiently motivated by a greater sense of control and direction over its own affairs, find the resources to provide INSET activities according to its own particular needs." (Hewton, 1988, p 7)

Its advocates claimed that if professional development was school-based, that is occurring within the school itself, then the process of identifying needs would be easier, programmes could be more closely matched to those needs and the barriers to change would disappear. Choices about the content and delivery of such programmes would rest with teachers in schools.

This approach, like the course-based model, has severe limitations. It tends to under-estimate how sophisticated a task the identification of development needs usually is. It also fails to recognise that the management of change in schools is a complex process which often requires external as well as internal support. Further-more worries will arise that the professional development of the school is taking precedence over the personal development of the individual teacher. Also if a school draws exclusively on its own resources for professional development purposes, there is a danger of parochialism since no school can ever be in a situation where it has nothing to learn from those outside its immediate confines. There are also resource implications since this approach to professional development is,

> "... expensive in human resources and cash; and thus the potential effectiveness of the school-based model becomes a function of size; school-based INSET is likely to be richer in a large secondary school than in a small and relatively isolated primary school." (Henderson, 1979, p 19)

The school-focused model of professional development emerged as an attempt to modify the school-based model while retaining its essential school-based nature. The James Report on Teacher Education and Training set out a clear rationale for this approach. It emphasised more teacher involvement in planning the INSET activities and the incorporation of INSET into a schools broader strategy for development and improvement.

> "In-Service training should begin in the schools. It is here that learning and teaching take place, curricula and techniques are developed and needs and deficiencies revealed. Every school should regard the continued training of

its teachers as an essential part of its task, for which all members of staff share responsibility. An active school is constantly reviewing and re-assessing its effectiveness and is ready to consider new methods, new forms of organisation and new ways of dealing with the problems that arise." (DES, 1972, p 11)

Subsequently, Hoyle (1973) argued that INSET could best help in these areas if it was linked to specific school innovations, focused on functioning groups (eg, a departmental team or whole staff), backed by external support, including consultancy services from advisers and teachers' centres. He also proposed that schools should establish their own staff development programmes. This approach soon became known as the "school-focused" approach to professional development. It puts its emphasis upon planning INSET activities in relation to specifically identified innovations, intended developments, tasks and needs in a particular school. These activities may involve only a single teacher, a group of staff or the whole staff. They may be conducted either at the school site itself (school-based) or at external centres such as colleges or teachers' centres. It has three main elements: the identification of professional development needs, the implementation of appropriate programmes to meet those needs and the evaluation of the effectiveness of those programmes.

To some extent, this model took its momentum from the debate about the entitlement of teachers to programmes of professional development which was re-kindled by the discussion in the James Report (DES, 1972). James argued that the in-service professional development of teachers should be regarded as the third cycle of teacher training and that this should be as much a part of teacher education as is initial training. The report also argued for the identification in schools of senior members of staff who would act as professional development tutors to their colleagues and who would contribute to the coherent and long-term planning of professional development in the school. Had these developments taken place, choice would indeed have been in the hands of the practitioners. Access to full-time programmes of professional development has never been established in the way envisaged by James. Nor, until very recently, did many schools find the resources to undertake school focused professional development or to identify a senior member of staff as professional development tutor or co-ordinator. Instead the school focused model of professional development exhibited many of the weaknesses of the approaches. It sometimes degenerated into a "tool kit" form of development where immediate problems were identified and short term remedies applied. It also failed to reconcile satisfactorily the development needs of the different levels in the schools. In short, with a few notable exceptions, this approach to professional development was not firmly embedded in school policy and did not receive the resources that it required in order to be successful. Thus, again, the complexities of initiating and sustaining change in schools was under estimated. Such changes could not successfully be implemented by single individuals or small groups unless they were firmly rooted in the overall policies of the school. Yet the school focussed approach provided no effective means of achieving this, except on a random basis. To be effective, therefore, the professional development of teachers needs to be embedded in whole-school policy in a systematic way.

Professional development and school policy

The conclusion that teacher's professional development needs to be closely linked with the policies of the school emerges clearly from the critique of the school-based and school-focused models. This third approach to professional development is based on the assumption that:
1. the development of teachers should be closely related to the overall planning and review processes of school management and
2. should take account of the various characteristics of staff and staff roles, as well as the characteristics of groups of teachers. This is sometimes called the task-led approach to professional development, but this term conveys a short-term, ad hoc, scheme of things with little coherent long-term planning, when the reverse is, in fact the case.

In Britain the policy-based professional approach to development first came to prominence in Education in Schools (DES, 1977) where we find that every teacher will be expected to benefit from professional development throughout his or her career,

> "in order to keep abreast of the subject, to extend and refine teaching techniques, to accommodate new patterns of school organisation, or to prepare for new responsibilities." (DES, 1977, p 29)

Did this mean that teachers were to be entitled to programmes of professional development? If so, what form would that entitlement take? Who would choose and what would be the available options?

In March 1983 the Department of Education and Science issued Circular 3/38, "The In-Service Training Grant Scheme." Few people at the time, especially among in-service providers, recognised how seminal a document this was to be. Within four years the provision of in-service training for teachers was to be radically re-organised and the nature of its funding changed significantly. As we have seen, in-service training was the province of institutions of higher education who provided an annual programme of long and short courses both nationally and within their own regions, usually in consultation with local education authorities (LEAs). Successful courses, those that were well attended, were repeated. Others were dropped or changed. Alternatively schools sought to develop their own programmes in relative isolation. Circular 3/38 was the first part of a process that was to change all this.

By 1985 it was being made explicit to all teachers that they were:

"expected to carry out their professional tasks in accordance with their judgment, without bias, precisely because they are professionals. This professionalism requires not only appropriate training and experience but also the professional attitude which gives priority to the interests of those served and is constantly concerned to increase effectiveness through professional development. The Government believes that this concern should be fully taken into account in the policies for the staffing of schools and the training, deployment and management of teachers ... the professionalism of teachers also involves playing a part in the corporate development of the school. HMI reports frequently refer to the importance of professional team work, where the teachers within a school agree together on the overall goals of the school, on the policies for the curriculum in the widest sense ..."

(DES, 1985, p 44)

However, the document Better Schools (DES, 1985) went on to point out that although annual expenditure on in-service training for teachers was ƒ 100 million, there is widespread agreement that these resources are not used to the best advantage. LEAs and schools have little incentive to satisfy themselves that a particular form of professional development represents good value for money. Insufficient attention is given to evaluating the extent to which teachers and schools benefit from training undertaken (DES, 1985).

In order to achieve a much more systematic approach to planning the professional development of teachers, the in-service training of teachers has, since April 1987, been organised and financed under the Local Education Authority Training Grant Scheme (LEATGS). DES Circular 6/86 set out the new scheme: the Secretary of State would decide annually on national priority areas for in-service training, and indicate the level of funding available to local education authorities. LEAs would submit their INSET proposals and those approved by the DES would qualify for grants of 70% towards the cost of national priority training, and 50% towards programmes defined as local but not national priorities. This document also indicated that all professional development activity supported through this scheme should be monitored by the LEA in order to discover how far it has contributed to more effective and efficient delivery of the education service.

The goal is to promote more systematic and purposeful planning of the professional development of all teachers. In most LEAs this is facilitated, in part, by the devolution of part of the professional development budget to schools, thus not only giving the power of choice to practitioners but also providing them with resources. This sum is often expressed in terms of pounds per teacher, and is usually about 10% of the LEA's total in-service budget. Each institution draws up a detailed proposal for its professional development programme based on an internal process of identifying needs and taking into account local and national priorities. Schools then bid for funds to the LEA, just as it, in turn, bids to the DES. Each school must indicate how teaching staff were consulted in the preparation of the proposal, how the bid develops from earlier experience, what evaluation has taken place of previous professional development work in the school and how the planned programme will be evaluated.

At the same time as schools were being provided with funds to organise at least some of their school-based in-service training, they were also being given time in which to train. With the establishment of training days as part of the School Teacher's Pay and Conditions of Service Order (DES, 1987), schools were given time to implement their own plans for professional development. The basic working year for teachers was deemed to consist of some 1265 hours, of which some time could be set aside for working parties and meetings. LEAs were allocated five training days when teachers could work together in the absence of children. Some of these days were used for national and local priorities, but others were allocated to schools for the professional development of their own staff.

Table 1. Models of professional development

APPRENTICESHIP MODEL

Advantages	Disadvantages	Assumptions
* immediacy * relevance * low cost * available in school * focus on individual needs * teachers can make choices	* no coherent needs analysis * may be ad hoc * needs may not be met * may not be developmental * focus *only* on individual needs	* that individuals can plan own development alone * that what is good for the individual teacher is good for the school * individuals can change schools

COURSE-BASED MODEL

* can increase knowledge and improve skills * teachers can make choices from what is offered * provides opportunity to reflect on professional practice * may be full-time * can lead to further qualifications * can enhance promotion prospects	* may be too theoretical * choices determined by providers * may not reflect school needs * may not have practical application in the classroom * ignores teacher expertise * may be high cost * may require long time commitment	* one teacher can influence whole school or groups of colleagues * theory can be translated into practice by teacher * a wide variety of different needs can be met by the same course

Bell ❖❖

Table 1. continued
SCHOOL-BASED / SCHOOL-FOCUSED MODEL

Advantages	Disadvantages	Assumptions
*based on school needs * schools can provide own programme * enables schools to use outside expertise * may cope with different levels of professional development * can use teacher expertise	* requires ability to identify needs clearly * some schools may not have sufficient expertise or resourses * may lead to parochialism * may lead to concentration on remedial or top-up approach leading to a lack of coherence * may undervalue individual needs while over emphasising school needs	* that all schools can identify own needs * that schools have sufficient resourses to meet needs * professional development will be linked to whole school policies

PROFESSIONAL DEVELOPMENT MODEL

* is an overall approach to school development * enables schools to choose appropriate methods of development * some resources are earmarked * external support is available * is subject to agreement of governors * priorities have to be identified	* insufficient resources may be available * may be overtaken by LEA or DES policy priorities * is subject to agreement of governors and to enfluence by LEAs * may lead to emphasis on school needs rather than those of individual teachers * can be seen as a challenge to teachers' professional autonomy * may be linked to appraisal	* that medium and long term planning is possible * policy, once formulated, can be implemented in classrooms * resources will be made available * whole school policies are the most effective approach to managing and improving schools

We find, therefore, that teachers at all levels in the school expected to avail themselves of professional development opportunities. They are also expected to take part in helping to provide such opportunities for colleagues. Furthermore, the nature of the resourcing for professional development now makes it more likely that individual teachers, groups of teachers and teachers acting as a whole school, may have a direct part to play in formulating the professional development policy for their school. In the words of Circular 6/86,

"The Secretary of State will wish to assure himself that these proposals are related to systematically assessed needs and priorities are set within balanced and coherent overall policies and plans and built appropriately on the strength of current arrangements." (DES, 1986, p 7)

In order to achieve this, schools require a mechanism for establishing aims and a co-ordinating mechanism for ensuring that groups and individuals work together towards agreed objectives. The effect of this approach is to shift the arena within which choices about professional development are made to the interface between the school and the LEAS. It also gives a much more proactive role to the practitioner in the school who now may do more than express preferences from a range of available options. The practitioner is now more able to determine the form of professional development that is offered to colleagues within one or a group of schools based on the time and money that is available for that purpose. Teachers in schools can play a part in identifying their own professional development needs although tensions still remain between the legitimate demands of individuals for personal development and the policy needs of the school. Furthermore, the impact on the school and its teachers of making one choice rather than another becomes much more real. Thus if the choice in one school is for a full-term secondment for one teacher and a full-day's training for every teacher, the choice, while not easy, is clear.

This shifting of the arena within which choices are made has not been without difficulties. For example, there is still evidence to suggest that professional development programmes are managed in a relatively arbitrary way, and take little heed of the long term needs of the school and of individuals within the school (Cowan and Wright, 1990). The in-service days which are the major part of current professional development strategies of many schools and LEAs undoubtedly have enhanced the ability of practitioners to make choices and to meet their own needs. One recent investigation concluded that in-service days:

"- encouraged better staff co-operation
– encouraged better use of facilities
– has led to improved strategies for all school systems, discipline, resources
– helped to establish school appraisal scheme
– provided time to exchange ideas
– created opportunities to visit, liaise with colleagues in other departments and institutions
– helped school develop policies
– raised staff awareness
– helped to highlight specific needs."
    (Cowan and Wright, 1990, p 117)

At the same time, however, the same training days:
– failed to match the needs of the school as a whole;

- did not ensure that individual needs are met;
- were not usually evaluated by staff to ensure both an avoidance of mistakes next time and continuing commitment from staff to any plans or policies formulated;
- occurred at times which were inappropriate or which made immediate follow-up impossible;
- were not based on long-term professional development plans;
- had themes which often occurred in isolation and without regard for previous or subsequent activities.

(derived from Cowan and Wright, 1990)

These criticisms remind us of the importance of locating professional development within an overall policy framework. This model is in its infancy in Britain and Wales and there is still some way to go before its success or failure can be established. It is based on the assumption that professional development as an integral part of whole-school policy will be effective both as part of the continuing process of managing the school and as a contributory factor in initiating and supporting necessary changes. Such an approach allows professional development to be systematically planned and resourced as a part of an overall school development plan. This is the essence of the Developmental Model of Teacher Professional Development. It is based on a coherent set of policies for school improvement and it places the professional development of the staff in the school at the centre of those policies as a crucial element in providing an even more worthwhile education for the children. It also provides the practitioner with increased opportunities for choice and, at the same time, places upon the same practitioner burdensome responsibilities for managing the professional development process. A discussion of some of these responsibilities will form a major part of the next section, as will an examination of some of the implications for LEAs and institutions of higher education in their role as providers of professional development programmes.

Some implications of practitioner choices in professional development

As a result of the changes in emphasis in the ways of providing for the professional development of teachers, it is possible to identify a range of implications. In this final section, I intend to focus on three main sets of issues. These are:

1. The implications for schools as they try to come to terms with managing their professional development activities and incorporate those activities into a coherent school development plan.
2. The implications for LEAs, especially their inspector and advisor teams as their role changes from providers to facilitators and evaluators of professional development.

3. The implications for institutions of higher education, especially universities, as they seek to develop relevant short courses and consultancies.

Some implications for schools

The Education Reform Act (1988) now makes it mandatory for every school with over 200 pupils to manage its own budget. This devolving of financial management to schools is colloquially known as Local Management of Schools (LMS). It is based on the quaint Thatcherite assumption that all management is financial management. While the LEA remains in control of the professional development budget the school can now use its own resources to supplement what it receives from the LEA. It may look at a wide range of alternative providers in order to meet its professional development needs. It also has to produce a school development plan which shows how it intends to implement the new National Curriculum and how it will meet the many other challenges of the 1990s. This plan has, at its centre, the continued development of the teachers in the school.

Choices about the professional development of teachers must be located in the overall policy for the development of the school. To achieve this the school development plan must contain a clear view about how teacher development can contribute to the implementation of that plan. The implication of this is that the development plan will be constructed with the aims of the school fore front as its main point of reference. We can see from Figure 1 below that the construction of such a plan is in fact a cyclical process involving eight stages. For practitioners to make informed choices about professional development for individual teachers, groups of teachers or for the whole school, the plan, and especially the resource allocation stage, must take full account of how staff resources need to be managed in order to achieve the target outcomes. All staff in the school must be aware of the key elements of the school's development plan and be able to recognise how

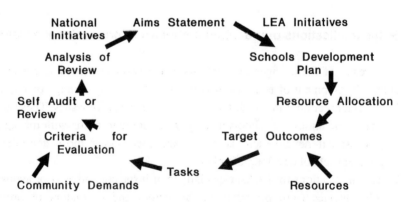

Figure 1. The school development plan (derived from Bell, 1991)

they can make a contribution to it. What, then, is a school development plan and how is it produced?

A school development plan is a flexible instrument to support the management of the school. It is a cyclical process, not a finished product and operates over a three year period with targets for the first year being very specific, those for the second year less so and only broad indications of intent given for year three. There are several essential features of the planning process:

- The school needs to have an aims statement which identifies the essential purpose of the school and guides all those in the school as they carry out their various duties. This will have to be a succinct, practical statement rooted in what the school is already doing rather than based on some vague philosophy or on some unattainable ideal.
- The school will have to know what it is already doing and how well it is functioning. It will require, therefore, a regular process of self-review or audit.
- As a result of analysing this audit priorities can be established for the next phase of development planning and, if necessary, the aims statement can be revised.
- The plan, when constructed, will identify a manageable number of development targets and establish a timescale for meeting them. It will also show how resources, including finance, time and the professional development of all the staff of the school will be organised to help achieve the targets in the development plan.
- These will be further sub-divided into target outcomes or precise objectives together with a clear indication of how and by when they are to be achieved.
- The target outcomes will be expressed in terms of tasks to be performed by particular people within the school, perhaps working with colleagues from outside the school such as consultants, inspectors or advisers.
- Criteria for evaluating how far the tasks have been achieved, resources adequately and appropriately deployed and professional development programmes effectively carried out will be built in to the plan. These criteria and the evaluation which is based on them will then form the starting point for the next audit. One of the most significant features of this stage will be the evaluation of the teachers' professional development programme, since staff development is crucial if the plan is to be successful.

We can see from Figure 1 that the plan is not to be constructed in the school in isolation from other factors. Initiatives from elsewhere in the education system will impinge on the planning as well: the availability of resources and demands of parents and the priorities of the members of the school's wider community. This process is in its very early stages in schools. Already it is having a profound effect on the professional development choices that practitioners make and on the ways in which they make those choices. Professional development is now beginning to be seen as a major management responsibility to the extent that all schools have at least one senior member of staff responsible for it. In larger schools, often a team of teachers working together on identifying needs and organising programmes. As a result of this, however, those with responsibility for the professional development of colleagues are recognising the need for further training and support, especially in the areas of identifying professional development needs and in planning programmes. Thus one set of implications for giving practitioners the power of choice in professional development is that further professional development is required in order to ensure that choice is exercised for the benefit of the whole school within the framework of its development plan. An important part of this further training is the skill necessary to identify professional development needs.

A research project (Carter and Bell, 1986) designed to identify appropriate ways of establishing what the professional development needs of teachers were and how they could be related to school needs concluded that the two key features for the successful identification of professional development needs by teachers were:

a. openness and clear communication and

b. the opportunity for practitioners to take ownership of the process, whatever form that process took.

It was also suggested that any formal or structured process of identifying professional development needs must start from a common point at which all staff can share an understanding of what the process is and what its outcomes will be. It has to be decided whether the initial focus will be on identifying the needs of individuals or those of the school. Either starting point can make for a valid and useful contribution to the integration of professional development into an overall school development plan. Whatever the starting point, the process has to attempt the difficult task of reconciling individual, group and school needs. Figure 2, (derived from Carter and Bell, 1986) shows how one school began with a whole school training day which focused on the possible methods of identifying professional development needs. All staff were consulted about their own needs and those of the school. Individual needs were then explored further through a series of interviews with a staff group elected for that purpose. That group then made recommendations to the headteacher and the senior management team of the school about the range of individual development needs, and how they might best be prioritised to fit into the needs of departments, teams and of the whole school. The senior management team produced a draft school development plan, incorporating these ideas which was discussed by the whole staff in groups. As a result of the feedback from these discussions, a final version of the plan was produced by the head and her senior management team and sent to the governing body for discussion. This process has it drawbacks. It is cumbersome and time consuming. It requires several tasks to be carried out at least twice. It can never resolve all the

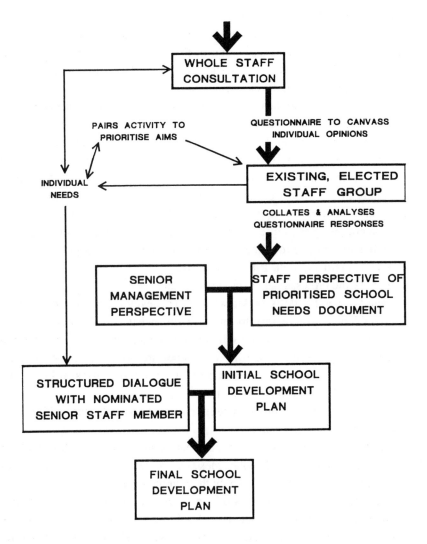

WHOLE STAFF
CONSULTATION

PAIRS ACTIVITY TO
PRIORITISE AIMS

QUESTIONNAIRE TO CANVASS
INDIVIDUAL OPINIONS

INDIVIDUAL
NEEDS

EXISTING, ELECTED
STAFF GROUP

COLLATES & ANALYSES
QUESTIONNAIRE RESPONSES

SENIOR
MANAGEMENT
PERSPECTIVE

STAFF PERSPECTIVE OF
PRIORITISED SCHOOL
NEEDS DOCUMENT

STRUCTURED DIALOGUE
WITH NOMINATED
SENIOR STAFF MEMBER

INITIAL SCHOOL
DEVELOPMENT
PLAN

FINAL SCHOOL
DEVELOPMENT
PLAN

Figure 2. External consultant input on school needs

inevitable conflicts. It did however produce a school development plan that is understood and, on the whole, accepted by the practitioners who see how their development needs fit into those of the school. They can also recognise those areas in which future development opportunities will exist in future. This helps some teachers with their career planning.

This approach to the identification of professional development needs for teachers tends to ignore some crucial areas that ought, at times, to be taken into account. For example, it may or may not include an analysis of job descriptions to ensure that all necessary duties are being carried out. It may or may not focus on the extent to which those responsibilities are being carried out effectively. This takes us into the area of staff appraisal which is a contentious issue at the moment (see Bell, 1988b, for a further discussion of this as it relates to professional development.) It is clear, however, that standards of performance must be a factor in identifying professional development needs.

Any analysis of professional development needs, presupposes that some, if not all, of those needs can and will be met. A further implication of practitioner choice in the field of professional development is that these needs can be met within the resources of the school, or through the resources of the LEA. More will be said about the role of the LEA in the next section and about the use of other providers, especially in the role of consultants, in the section after that. Within the school, however, practitioners require access to skills and knowledge to enable them to provide programmes to meet their own professional development needs and those of their colleagues. Providing programmes for staff development falls into six stages (Bungard and Bell, 1986). These are:

– Identify the professional development needs.
– Identify specific skills or knowledge. To develop further professional skills effectively it is necessary to know exactly what it is that colleagues need to know or be able to do, as a result of a professional development programme.
– Decide target population. All programmes are not suitable for all colleagues. This was a major criticism of externally provided courses. It has to be made clear for whom the course is intended.
– Set objectives for the programme in terms of what colleagues will be able to do as a result of the programme.
– Plan and implement the programme bearing in mind that professional development is most effective if colleagues acquire new skills in a practical way and just before they will need to apply them in their classrooms.
– Evaluate the programme at two levels. Firstly, how appropriate was it for the target group in terms of pace, level, usefulness and relevance and, secondly, in terms of how far the stated objectives were achieved. This latter form of evaluation may require some subsequent follow up as colleagues seek to apply new skills or knowledge.

Letting the practitioners choose, therefore, extends to more than making choices about the identification of professional development needs and selecting how they may be met. An inevitable consequence of practitioner choice is practitioner participation in the provision of programmes to meet identified needs. This process becomes more marked as schools accept more responsibility for their own development through the process of development planning and as more resources for carrying out the development of teachers acrue to the school. The LEA, however, still provides the policy framework within which development planning takes place. It still allocates resources on the basis of the bids that it receives from the practitioners in the schools. The LEAs' resources are determined, in turn, by the response of the DES to the bids that it receives from LEAs. It is to the management of these resources and the extent to which that process has been influenced by practitioner choice over the professional development process that we now turn.

The implications for local education authorities

The framework created by the new Local Education Authority Training Grant Scheme (LEATGS) devolves some funding for the professional develoment of teachers to the schools. There are also up to five training days available for use by schools. The DES has recognised the role of the LEAs in furthering national and local priorities. It has reminded LEAs, however, that programmes of professional development can serve the needs of teachers and lecturers from a single institution or from a group of institutions. LEA inspectors and advisors can be involved at every stage from the identification of needs to the evaluation and follow-up programmes.

The contribution of LEAs to the professional development of teachers was recently evaluated by *Her Majesties' Inspectors of Schools* (HMI). They found that the introduction of the LEATGS scheme has resulted in a more systematic approach to the planning, organisation and delivery of professional development programmes. In general terms, this work is now more healthy than it has been at any time previously. All LEAs have designated an inspector or adviser or officer with overall responsibility for INSET, but most of these new appointees have been given little or no training in preparation for their new role. This was a serious deficiency which is now being addressed by more LEAs as the scheme progresses. The people appointed to these posts tended to lead a management team with the overall responsibility for planning the LEAs professional development provision. It was clear (DES, 1989) that many of these teams lacked sufficient clerical and support staff to cope with the demands of the scheme. In general, schools have welcomed the opportunity to assume responsibility for the planning and delivery of a part of their overall professional development plan. This has released enormous energy and professionalism among teachers. There have been problems associated with the devolution of budgets. Institutions have not had access to the necessary training. Budgets are not always related to development plans agreed with the LEAs. The administrative burden on institutions has been considerable and the financial monitoring and information flow from LEAs has not always helped institutional planning. These problems now need to be confronted at both school and LEA levels in order that practitioners can make the most effective choices and so that LEAs can continue to make a significant input into all aspects of the professional development of teachers.

Advisory teachers working alongside colleagues in school have proved to be an effective way of meeting some of the immediate, classroom and curriculum-based needs of individual teachers. They have provided an effective form of professional development for departments, teams and even whole schools in areas such as Information Technology, primary school science and technology. Their existence has extended the range of practitioner choice. At the same time the LEATGS scheme which facilitated the expansion of such provision, has raised questions about the ownership of professional development provision. It has also required LEAs to set up appropriate structures to manage such provision. Significantly, however, those structures are just as concerned about the identification and articulation of the professional development needs of teachers in their schools as they are with the delivery of programmes. LEAs increasingly have to take into account school priorities as well as those that they have identified. Both schools and LEAs have to be aware of national priorities. It would be misleading to suggest that these three sets of priorities are always in conflict or that practitioners will not take them into account when making their own professional development choices. Nevertheless,

"... the tensions between individual, institutional and authority needs are of concern to many LEAs personnel and teachers, some believing that personal needs are increasingly being overlooked." (DES, 1989, p 6)

The implications for institutions of higher education as they extend their short course and consultancy work

The major impact of these changes in the approaches to the professional development of teachers on programme providers in higher education has been,

"a significant reduction in the number of teachers on full-time secondment for award-bearing courses ... Many institutions have responded to the need for greater flexibility and closer targeting of provision to need by modularising provision and accrediting LEA and school-based INSET." (DES, 1989, p 5)

This situation has been exacerbated by the extent to which LEAs have devolved funds for professional development to schools. The effect of this has been to provide schools with sufficient resources to enable a significant number of teachers to benefit from short courses or a very limited number to attend long, award-bearing programmes. Schools also have to target professional development funding so, short courses are generally preferred. Now that schools can use training days and can also fund courses specially designed to meet their own needs, providers are now likely to find themselves working in very close collaboration with single schools, groups of schools, or targeted schools within an LEA. This relationship, unlike the traditional provider-receiver relationship within professional development programmes, is characterised by:

- teachers in schools identifying needs;
- schools or LEAs having resources to meet own priorities;
- potential, client schools or LEAs negotiating with a range of possible providers;
- providers being required to show how they would meet needs identified by clients;
- clients bidding for the opportunity to provide programmes based on negotiated contract;
- choice residing with client.

In short, the provision of professional development programmes is moving towards a form of client (teacher/school/LEA) – consultant (provider) relationship where the need, or problem to be addressed is defined within the school and is then addressed by the provider/consultant. This relationship between the client and consultant can take a variety of forms. It might be based on advocacy where the consultant takes a particular position relative to a problem and seeks to have his view adopted by the client. It might also include the role of change agent who assists in diagnosing and planning for some change focusing on the process rather than goals or outcomes. This typology (summarized in table 2) suggests that the roles of both expert and facilitator are appropriate at different times.

The consultant as expert

The role of consultant as expert is based on the assumption that the expert consultant has knowledge and skills which the client does not have. Added to this is the related assumption that the client will never need or want to have such skills or knowledge. The client purchases the necessary skills from an expert external to his organisation to having firstly identified, defined and specified the problem to which he requires a solution. The expert consultant is expected to accept as given the client's definition of the problem, and the client's assumption that a solution of the problem is possible, and that it can be identified and implemented. This requires that the consultant is a problem-solving expert who can provide either an acceptable solution or a set of viable alternatives on the basis of a command of expert knowledge.

As resources become available for using consultants as providers of professional development in schools, it is questionable whether or not the will to use them can be found. Many teachers would argue that if a consultant cannot tell them what to do in their class- rooms to solve their immediate problems, then he or she should not be working in schools. They might also argue that the consultant is so remote from the closed world of those very classrooms that s/he cannot possibly have any relevant expertise. Should it be discovered that this was not the case there may even be teachers who could and would see the work of a consultant as a challenge or threat to their own professionalism. They may well fail to implement recommendations or do so in an indifferent way. Educational change has many examples of such innovations coming to grief in this way.

It is this very distinction between the expert and the client that provides the strengths and the weaknesses of this approach to consultancy. The expert is an outsider and therefore not involved in the organisational politics of the school. Although s/he is associated with the management of the institution, the consultant is, in some senses, neutral since there exists a clear contractual relationship with the client organisation. On the other hand such a specific division between client and consultant tends to mytho- logise the role which consultants play. It requires that many independent factors combine effectively for the relationship to work. The client obviously believes that more knowledge will either solve the problem or meet the need as perceived or facilitate necessary change. The consultant has generated the expectation that he or she can, at least, contribute to this process. The whole relationship between client and consultant is based on the assumption that it is the problem or need which the client has identified that requires to be solved. The consultant is not expected to ask why that particular problem has been identified. It can be argued, therefore, that this type of client-consultant relationship is firmly based on the philosophy and assumptions of utilitarianism.

Such consultancy assumes that change within schools is based on a notion of rationality according to which people will respond in the required way on the basis of new information. In such a situation the consultant only has to provide an appropriate development programme, and rational people will change in the appropriate way. Truth, as the consultant, and perhaps also the client, see it, is vested with power to change. Prejudice, inefficiency, sectional self-interest, malpractice and a whole variety of other organisational ills can thus be affected by the skilled consultant who presents the client and the client's organisation with the relevant truths. Once the individuals within the organisation are exposed to this new information they, and therefore the organisation, will respond by changing. Stated in such a bald manner this appears to be a caricature of the client-consultant relationship. Yet it does indicate some of the basic premises on which that relationship is founded and upon which it might flounder.

The consultant as facilitator

The consultant as facilitator tends not to be an expert in some field related to the technical or structural aspects of the organisation's activity. This non-directive form of consultancy normally focuses on the process aspect of activity rather than specific task achievement. The mode of intervention focuses on the interpersonal aspects of an organisation's activity. It is assumed that once this is managed effectively changes will occur in other parts of the structure. The organisational difficulties with which this work deals are all approached as if they result from a lack of interpersonal communication, a lack of shared power or ineffective use of delegation or some other similar interactional problem. The consultant's role is to encourage and to facilitate relevant changes in these areas perhaps through the provision of programmes to develop appropriate skills. Such interventions are not undertaken as an isolated event, concentrating on one subsection of the organisation's activity. They are intended to make an impact on the organisation as a total system. This view of the organisation as total system is current in most of such intervention strategies which do not necessarily concentrate on immediate problems. Facilitative consultancy not only sees these problems as central to total problem-solving for the school. It also seeks to establish within the institution the facility to anticipate and solve other problems of the future.

This type of client-consultant relationship flows from collaborative problem definition, and collaborative attempts at finding solutions. The diagnosis and the planning are carried out co-operately, in order to obtain commitment to them and their implementation. The change strategies developed by this co-operative process and put into operation during the action stage of the consultancy are assumed to be a smooth process because commitment has been generated. As a result of these collaborative activities the client will be able to develop the necessary skills to identify and solve problems as they may emerge. It has to be recognised that this client-consultant relationship, like that based on expert knowledge, is a temporary one. However, the processes involved are intended to create a permanent improvement in the functioning of the school. It is the very adherence to values such as co-operation, collaboration, openness and power equalisation that is intended to bring about such changes.

Table 2. Consultant as expert and/or facilitator

Expert	Facilitator
Knowledge or skills based	Process based
emphasis is on Problem Solution	emphasis is on Problem ownership
relates to Management	relates to Whole Staff
clear division of roles consultant and client	consultant and client co-operate
assumes rational processes of change	assumes that change is generated by and through personal interaction
sees schools as a system	sees school as a collection of individuals who are loosely interdependent
evaluation focuses on outcomes	evaluation focuses on processes

The client needs to be aware of how the consultant is attempting to bring about organisational change, and the value assumptions which are being made about the desirability of such things as free communication, openness and honesty. These values in some situations, run counter to those espoused by many of the teachers who wish to conduct their professional activities within the enclosed world of the four walls of the classroom. A clash of values may ensue from the introduction of such a consultant. For change to take place throughout the school the facilitative consultant must be able to assume that the school operates as a loosley coupled social system. The school is seen as a collection of subsystems connected in such a way that various changes in one area will automatically produce changes in others. Schools must display or be helped to develop collaborative forms of openness, adaptability and commitment to change for this approach to work. The client needs to recognise this, and has to be sure that the disruption and conflict which may follow will, in fact, have the required pay-off in terms of an improvement in the performance of the school and in the quality and effectiveness of teaching and learning inside the school.

The client-consultant relationship is a problem-centred, temporary one. Once the problem has been tackled the consultant has to withdraw, having avoided the establishing of a relationship in which the client is too dependent on the consultant whether for expertise or process skills. Thus the relationship between the consultant and client is essentially a marginal one. Both sides have to recognise and take account of this marginality. The consultant is in but not of the school. He or she may have support from some members of it, but others are likely to see the consultant as threatening. There will, for each type of consultant, be a discrepancy between his or her values and those of the client school. This will mean that, whatever change method is used, the consultant will become involved in a series of conflicting relationships which will serve to emphasise this marginality. The client often fails to recognise this element in the relationship. Within any form of consultancy or helping relationship, therefore, a whole range of issues arise both for the client and the consultant. Within such a relationship there is a need on both sides for the recognition that not only do certain objectives have to be achieved, but also certain types of relationships established. Within the helping situation all parties need to feel some ability to exercise power and to develop other types of affiliations. Trust in the client-consultant relationship is an important commodity. Since, in most cases, trust is based on understanding and understanding is based on knowledge, the most effective set of guidelines which can be given to a client in a school who wishes to use a consultant is, first to know your requirement and then to know your consultant.

In order to understand fully what a consultant can and cannot do in schools we need to take account of the extent to which the consultant is required to provide professional development based on the identification and meeting of clients' needs. Professional development in schools is increasingly becoming demand-led rather than supply-led. As a consequence the consultant who becomes part of the in-service programme of a school has to ensure that professional development needs are properly identified. The expertise and structures must be in place to enable those needs to be met. It is the involvement of teachers in the identification of their own professional development needs that helps to generate a sense of ownership of the development process. It is the extent to which those needs are met either by the teachers themselves, or by other teachers working as trainers, or by outside consultants which will give credibility to the process.

The extent to which universities and other institutions of higher education are having to respond in a consultancy mode to the provision of professional development programmes for teachers is leading to a fundamental re-consideration of some of the more traditional activities of those institutions. Not only are they being required to re-think what they provide, how they provide it, and how these programmes are accredited. They are also having to re-conceptualise the nature and purposes of educational research.

Consultancy as research

Research normally consists of some form of investigation of a defined problem or issue with the intention of achieving an outcome that may well have no practical application but that can eventually be made public in a written form. Even within this extremely broad formulation, consultancy, even consultancy grounded in research, tends to be marginalised as research activity. It is a mistake, however, to assume that research is, in fact, a unified or a unifiable set of activities using an agreed methodology and leading to identifiable findings that can be made public. Research might best be understood as a series of choices, the first of which will be about the nature of the research itself and how it is initiated. Ziman (1988), for example, has argued that research might be either "curiosity-directed" or "results-oriented". The first of these involves the pursuit of ideas for their own sake. Goals or outcomes, if they exist, belong only to the researcher and there is no pressure to produce instant results or direct applications. The second approach to research takes the form of the pursuit of answers to sponsor-defined problems where the sponsor may identify the parameters within which the research takes place and within which the answers or solutions may be formulated. We do not have here two mutually exclusive alternative approaches to research, only one of which falls within the acceptable tradition. In fact, Ziman identifies two approaches to research each with its own traditions and expectations and each having its own place in the totality of research activity. This is what I have termed the Dual Economy Paradigm of Educational Research (see table 3). Curiosity-directed research emphasises ideas and problems; is concerned with methodology and originality and is not concerned with 'real-world' applications. Results-oriented

Table 3. The dual-economy paradigm of research

CURIOSITY – DIRECTED RESEARCH	RESULTS – ORIENTED RESEARCH

Emphasis on:
  ideas
  problems
  issues
	Emphasis on:
	  outcomes
	  solutions
	  practical applications

Concern with:
  quality
  originality
  accessibility
  methodological
    soundness
	Concern with:
	  applications
	  relevance
	  cost effectiveness
	  financial returns
	  results

Not concerned with:
  results
  deadlines
  financial returns
  'real world' applications
	Not concerned with:
	  ideas
	  problems
	  issues

RESEARCHER INSPIRED AND FOCUSED	MARKET OR SPONSORING AGENCY DIRECTED AND FOCUSED

research emphasises outcomes and solutions and is concerned with results and applications rather than with abstract ideas and theoretical issues. The former may well be researcher inspired and focused, while the latter will be sponsoring agency focused and controlled.

Curiosity-based research has two main strands, the positive and the interpretive. The former, as Ribbins (1986) argues, is based on conjecture and refutation and moves by deduction from the general to the particular. The latter is based on conjecture and explanation and moves by induction from the particular to the general. These approaches share one characteristic in common. They both appear to be made up of a series of discrete and linear stages. This may not be an entirely accurate depiction for the process of data collection and data interpretation are closely inter-related in interpretive studies. Interpretative studies which also tend to concentrate to a far greater extent than positivistic work on attempting to understand and explain how schools actually work and how they are perceived by those within them.

In the results-oriented research, similarly, we find a number of distinctive strands. Much of such work in the British education system tends either to be evaluative or consultancy-based. In evaluation-based research, the agenda for the research may be a product of the pre-existing context and will be determined by what is to be evaluated and for whom the evaluation is being conducted. Evaluation itself, where it is funded by external bodies, takes the form of intensive and planned data collection on which informed judgments about policy implementation can be based. The significant feature of evaluative work is that it is not objective in the sense that it is more located in the political, social and ideological arenas than most other forms of research. In fact it takes us, "... deep into the areas in which policy, practice and research collide." (Bell, 1986, p 75) To the extent that the evaluation is formative rather than summative it can also involve the researcher in providing support for implementing the recommendations made as a result of the evaluation. The evaluator thus may become part of the situation being evaluated, rather than apart from it. The boundary between research and evaluation becomes blurred and the ownership of the outcomes may be unclear, but the outcome may be that the researcher/evaluator becomes an integral part of the professional development of the practitioners whose work is being evaluated.

Such issues also emerge in consultancy-based research. Here it is the client who creates the initial frame of reference, often independently of the consultant. The agenda will be a product of the client's analysis of the situation and of what the consultant can bring to it. Thus client expectations and knowledge are central to the process. As we have seen, the ownership of the consultancy process may remain with the consultant, but the client may well wish to influence its application The ownership of the outcomes will usually remain with the client although, again, there may be an obligation on the part of the consultant to implement at least some of the recommendations. Consultancy thus moves into an area where issues of definition and ownership can be significantly problematic yet it can also take research into areas which other forms of research cannot reach. Much depends on the shared expectations about the nature of consultancy which exists between consultant and client.

Concerns such as these emerge as a central part of the process of providing and supporting the professional development of teachers. Universities as providers have to address such issues and explore with colleagues in schools, LEAs and other providing agencies how the roles of provider-as-consultant and provider-as-researcher can be encompassed within the existing framework of research activity and, to what extent the boundaries of that framework have to become extended in order to contain a growing and increasingly important sphere of activity; that of supporting the professional development of teachers in ways determined by practitioner choice rather than provider direction.

Conclusion

Practitioners in schools have always been able to make choices about their own professional development. These choices have been both constrained and informed by the context within which they have had to be made and by the perspectives that practitioners have adopted in making them. Teachers whose main perspective was derived from their own classroom practice and related to their own career progression would tend to have a perspective on development that was significantly different from that of somebody with responsibility for managing a team of teachers. In a similar way the perspective adopted by senior management in a school, while recognising the validity of the other two perspectives, would tend to reflect a concern for the whole school rather than only for isolated parts of it.

The choices that are made available to practitioners, in turn, are shaped by prevailing notions of what, legitimately, might be regarded as appropriate forms of professional development. Apprenticeship is perfectly acceptable model under some circumstances but there are many things that cannot be achieved in this way. The course-based model provides valuable opportunities for individual professional development but there are considerable doubts as to whether this should be the only or even the predominant model for professional development if the intention is to improve and extend the quality of teaching and learning that is made available to children in our schools. School-based professional development can create an ethos within a school for the successful management of school-based change but it might also prove to be restrictive and parochial in the longer term. In a similar way the school-focused model can lead to a series of short term remedial activities or to a problem solving approach that does not facilitate the long-term, planned development of the school. All of these models offer different opportunities for practitioner choice and practitioner control over professional development.

Development through learning is central to everything that is done in schools in the name of education. This must be as true of the teachers as it is of the pupils. It must also be true of the organisation itself. The creation of an organisation that can sustain its own growth and development must now become the single most important purpose of practitioner professional development. This does not necessarily mean that teachers will have no choice but to subjugate their individual professional development needs to those of the school, although it does mean that priorities have to be established.

The policy-based model of professional development that is now emerging does offer an opportunity to practitioners to extend their control over their own development, albeit within a framework of provision and resourcing that is closely related to the needs of the school and to the development plan that formulates and expresses those needs. This plan can ensure that the most effective use is made of the expertise acquired by individuals as part of their professional development. At the same time, it provides a mechanism by which the needs and priorities of groups can be related to those of the whole school. Only in this way can the competing choices of those at different levels in the organisation be reconciled within a framework that allows practitioners to make informed choices about professional development programmes.

Chapter 5

TRANSFERRING PRACTITIONER RESEARCH

Hugo Letiche, Erasmus University Rotterdam & Amsterdam Polytechnic

Introduction

In this chapter I address the problem of transferring Practitioner Research from centres of established usage to target groups with little (without) prior experience in its use. First I examine *What is it that is to be transferred*; and then *How is this to be done?* Practitioner Research is: *What the target group is supposed to do*; scenarios will be developed to examine *How to get the target group to do it.* My assumptions are:

(1) Furthering the implementation of Practitioner Research depends neither on developing new forms of action, nor on providing new argumentation for that action, but on effectively utilizing and adapting known models (see Nias, Day, Handal, Bell).

(2) Practitioner Research can be conceptually understood as a *system* for describing work situations in order to better know, evaluate and improve on them; i.e. as a deliberate effort to influence teachers to adopt a critical voice with which to report and reflect on – most often in order to change – in-service experience.

(3) The successful transferring of Practitioner Research from existing centres-of-excellence to new initiatives depends on stakeholder response. Stakeholder response, in turn, depends on the success (or failure) of forging links between the social/philosophical presuppositions (ideology) implicit to practitioner research and the presuppositions (which they may or may not be aware of) of the stake-holders.

In the first section of the chapter I will analyze Practitioner Research into its component parts: (a) DESCRIPTIONS OF PRACTICE (b) ENTITLEMENT to speak out, (c) the COGNITIVE SKILLS needed for in-practice investigation, and

(d) the INTERACTIVE PRINCIPLES of a Practitioner / Facilitator relationship (see figure 1). I will give as generic a description of the phenomena as I can. In the second section I will explore several scenarios for transferring Practitioner Research be it successfully or unsuccessfully and examine the roles therein of crucial stake-holders and of their presuppositions.

The component parts of practitioner research

The component parts are the building blocks of practitioner research. While a rich variety of alternative forms of practitioner research exists, teachers as researchers ask and answer questions about professional (teaching / training / consulting) life in different and even competing ways, the combination of the component parts into one conceptual model will not (as is shown below) reduce lived complexity to theoretical neatness.

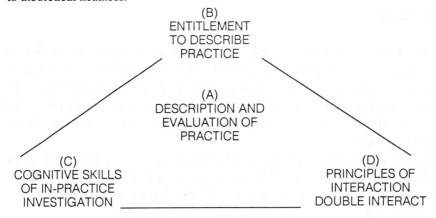

Figure 1

Description and evaluation

At the heart of the conceptual model one finds the description and evaluation of in-practice reality. This central idea is not easy to define; it is the result of the force field which the terms found in the three corners of the model (entitlement, cognitive skills and the principles of interaction) generate. These three elements are described later, after this initial discussion of the description of practice. The structure of the relationships and links between the three elements will be clarified first in order to reveal the characteristics of the central term. The constituent parts of Practitioner Research will thus be examined in a process of progressive differentiation.

The most general and inclusive definition is: *In practitioner research a practitioner DESCRIBES his/her in-service reality, criticizes this description, and examines the value to practice of the critique.*

The process of practitioner research hinges on the practitioner achieving an uncompromising honesty in expressing what s/he sees of in-service experience. It is important to appreciate what a burden it is to take critical repossession of one's own professional experience. Experience when purged of habit and routine looses its factitiousness and becomes turbulent and confusing. The effort to bring as much as possible of in-service activity to the level of awareness, needs encouragement and support, if it is to succeed. Practitioner Research demands that teachers write about and reflect on what they experientially know. Writing is so important because it is itself a stimulating, constructive thinking process. (Flower, 1985) While spoken language adheres to immediate circumstance, written language transforms it. Thought remains in speech the captive of immediate consciousness trapped in a paralysing transparency with circumstance. Spontaneous utterance is in-the-world; it is part and parcel of everyday circumstance. Speech is most often inseparable from what it outs, which frequently are the frustrations and habits of daily practice.

A written description of practice can only be produced when circumstance is conceptualized, i.e. put into a structured statement. This translation of circumstance into prose is a difficult process. Many practitioners do not like to write. They find the process of ordering and conceptualizing difficult and time consuming. The practitioner, if s/he is going to describe practice in writing, has to render in-service experience into text. A written description presents reality ordered, most often by means of systematic, hierarchical interrelationships. Writing is not simply saying what we mean; writing produces a processed version of thought. The individual stream of consciousness is very different from a readable text. Thus, description written by the practitioner to and for him/herself is cognitively different from speech. To write one has to compose; i.e. to decide in an act of transmission how to order one's material. Writing is a deliberate, purposeful form of expression; speech is often an intuitive outing of gut reaction.

Any circumstance can be described in a variety of ways. Descriptions of one and the same situation, made by colleagues, will vary. There will be diverging interpretations, a variety of emotional responses, dissimilar normative judgments. A description of the same event made at another time, or in another situation, will also be different. Description forces us to realize that existence isn't limited to one immediate, unquestionable present. The circumstances could be different, other choices might be made. The immediate, self-evident world of speech is replaced by the conceptual, modifiable world of writing.

A written description of in-service circumstance is produced only if the will to articulate context is strong enough. If the practitioner considers the process of putting practice into language to be significant for further professionalization, organizational development, or beneficial to his/her situation, then s/he will think about putting experience onto paper. The converting of in-service experience into written description transforms personal consciousness into an interpreted structured rendering of circumstance. It is in the nature of writing that a complex relationship is created between:

(a) the experiencing subject,

(b) the text,

(c) the original circumstance.

Reality is objectified; an internal and an external position are generated. On a first level, an experiencing *I* becomes a textual (described) *me*; on a second level, the *I* reads the text and is confronted with the *me*. The narrative assumes the first and second levels – circumstance and distance. It includes three elements: a doer, a speaker and a reader. One always writes for someone, for an assumed reader; in practitioner research one is one's own most important audience. Thus, only if convinced of the utilitarian value for oneself of representing in-service practice in narrative, will persons be willing to put in the time and effort needed to try to represent reality to themselves (in 'text') as it 'is'. Only after a situation has been rendered in writing, can it be questioned, radically doubted and evaluated.

Regrettably enough, there are very good reasons why practitioners find it so difficult to describe their work. Not only do the conditions surrounding the production of text have to be good (entitlement), but the potential practitioner researcher has to actually DO the work i.e. set him/herself the task of conceptualizing circumstance. To paraphrase a proverb: *You can bring the teacher to the classroom, but you can not force the practitioner to describe practice.* I assume that every social practice is in fact potentially describable, and know from experience that most social practice is for the persons directly involved indescribable. Practitioner research demands that persons transcend their signifying practices in order to generate descriptions. These descriptions can subsequently be (re-)examined to extract significance(s).

For the process of description and examination to succeed, practitioners often need support. The quality of investigation, I submit, depends most often on the soundness of interaction between the practitioner and facilitator. The quality of practitioner / facilitator interaction is examined later in this chapter.

Summarizing, we can see that there are two preconditions to practitioner research:

(1) practitioners have to be convinced that they possess an experience of in-service practice worth describing; and

(2) practitioners have to forge a (satisfactory) relationship in written language between themselves and their referent (context).

For practitioner research to occur, descriptions of practice have to be made which their author then criticizes. The teacher's conviction that it is valuable to describe his/her immediate context, I explore further as: *the achievement of ENTITLE-*

MENT; the means of making a qualitatively adequate written rendering of reality as: the *COGNITIVE SKILLS of in-practice investigation.* (Letiche, 1988a) And the contact between the practitioner and the facilitator is discussed as: the *Principles of INTERACTION.*

Entitlement

The teacher often needs, during the process of practitioner research, the stimulus of the Outsider's encouragement in order not to be overwhelmed by
(1) the flow of daily practice or
(2) the claims of experts that they have a monopoly on (scientific) knowledge.
It costs the practitioner a special effort to overcome the superficial assumptions of normalcy, i.e. to gain distance from the strangling web of in-service interactions. Two common, debilitating suppositions are:
(1) in practice there is nothing of import, and
(2) academic research methods represent for the practitioner an unattainable standard of excellence.
To overcome these barriers, the teacher-as-researcher has to be convinced that his/her practice is really worth studying from the insider's position. The *raison d'etre* of practitioner research is at issue. Is it really worthwhile to study one's own practice? After all practitioner experience often seems dull, merely life as usual. Professional practice may potentially involve rejoicing, boredom, embarrassment, complacency, pleasure, anger, self-pity, anxiety, and so on; but who actually sees all this?

> "The point is that almost everybody's business is to be occupationally ordinary ; that people take on the job of keeping everything utterly mundane ; that no matter what happens, pretty much everybody is engaged in finding only how it is that what is going on is usual, with every effort possible. And it is really remarkable to see people's efforts to achieve the 'nothing happened' sense of ...events" (Sacks, 1977).

For practitioner research to have a chance of success one has to be convinced that one is entitled to investigate in-service behaviour, conventions and thought.
Ordinary events have to be construed to have import, to be storyable. The practitioner has to see, that the way s/he does things is really tellable. In practitioner research the teacher observes professional behaviour, examines his/her interpretation of it, and shares this information. Such a task challenges anyone about to embark on it: Why is what you are going to describe, doubt, question important? *What entitles you to do research?* The practitioner will need to pay close attention to everyday, in-service activity; will need to attend to the commonplace and to witness the ordinary. Will practitioners believe that their experience is worth attending to? Can practitioners gain enough self-confidence,

that they will believe that *their* work is worthwhile or interesting enough to be studied? The answer to the question: What practice will be researched? depends on the reply to the quarry: Who is entitled to report on which experience(s)? Can and will practitioners find their own *voice*, and in an act of self-confirmation begin to do research on their own activity?

The problem for practitioner research is not one of methods, i.e. of designing suitable yardsticks for investigating practice; but is one of whether or not practitioners are going to decide that there is something worth knowing about their practice. The wherewithal to study everyday practice needs encouraging. Practitioners do not believe in the significance of their own experiencing; they must be encouraged to designate their actual circumstance as significant. In-service practice is too often seen to be ordinary: There's nothing special about it, i.e. Nothing ever happens here. This feeling, that one does not have a story to tell, is paramount to *doing ordinary*. In-service research depends on practitioners overcoming the prejudice that the everyday is banal, and recognizing the value of *voicing* their work experience.

The role of the facilitator is to encourage the practitioner to transcend doing ordinary and to discover his/her own *voice*. This task is paradoxical. On the one hand practitioners are to describe their circumstance, and on the other the description depends on a valuing of everyday reality which is at least in part created by the facilitator. The facilitator entitles practitioners to take their own experience seriously; s/he encourages them to see daily practice as interesting, important, tellable. Circumstance must not be lost in the nothing happened. (Weick, 1979) In the interaction between the Practitioner and the Facilitator the non-entitlement of doing ordinary is transformed into the limited entitlement necessary for doing research.

Cognitive skills of in-practice investigation

I agree with Jennifer Nias (in this volume) that the cognitive skills needed to do in-service research form a crucial source of practitioner learning which influence both research and teaching; but little analytical or empirical work has been done to clarify the nature of these skills, how they are transferred from pedagogue to practitioner, or the functioning of the interactions between learning, research and teaching. A way of thinking about the cognitive skills needed by the practitioner researcher, which I have found revealing, is to see him/her as inevitably *en procès*; which means (in French) to be *in the course of doing something* and *on trial*. (Kristeva, 1985) The nature of the cognitive skills of practitioner research is aptly summarized by this double-movement of being *en procès*. On the one hand the practitioner has to write up in-service events. Circumstance has to be brought into a symbolic system and integrated into a network of meanings to be describable. A narrative adhering to the dynamics of on-going and changing practice has to be generated. A report has to be made of what one does with the intent to examine and criticize practice on the basis of the description. On the other hand, practice is put on trial, i.e. one examines the quality of practice from a critical distance. In-service activity is seen from an external position, as if it belonged to another. The cognitive skills needed in the investigative process are those that both create a narrative of in-service reality and provide the necessary distance from in-practice occurrence.

What is meant by the first definition of *en procès*: to be in the course of doing things; what sort of things are practitioner researchers supposed to be doing? The successive stages to practitioner research are: I see something significant that is happening; I write-up what I see; I evaluate what I have written-up; I make plans to modify what I have understood; I take action; I see something significant that is happening; etc. Thus the first definition of *en procès* matches the action learning cycle. In practitioner research the teacher commences by re-representing reality in text. Writing is the tool for holding a mirror up to oneself. But this goal does not come easily. In talking with teachers and fellow facilitators I have discovered that it is very difficult to get teachers to write. (Lentz and Galesloot, 1988; Elliott, 1987) Practitioners do not identify writing with such things as: problem-solving, decision making or depth level learning. They see writing as a tedious task required of them (most often in a situation of accountability) by someone else. They write because they have to, not because they are convinced that it is functional for themselves. Writing is not perceived to be a way to think something through, nor a means to explore new possibilities. Writing is seen to be a way of being controlled, disciplined and administered. No wonder practitioners make use of safe, tried-and-true, formulas. Writing is a required representation of reality, for an audience who have some sort of power over one. A standard, rehearsed performance is the result. But in practitioner research writing is a strategic process that does not point to a pre-judged reality. Writing entails in principle:

> "[This] .. writing process (encompasses) ... a whole repertory of thinking processes such as planning, setting goals, generating new ideas, drawing inferences from old ideas, looking for relationships or patterns, and diagnosing problems and planning ways around them." (Flower, 1985)

To write effectively an active relationship has to be achieved between the writer and the text. During the composing process the teacher makes rough draft descriptions, generates tentative metaphors and makes exploratory associations: "writing is a mental three-ring circus." (Flower, 1985) The writer/researcher becomes (more) agile in conceiving and producing text. Writing sows the seeds of doubt – the practitioner sees the relativity of his/her truths when confronted with them on paper. The distancing effect of written language drives a wedge between the practitioner and immediate circumstance; it is this critical space which makes change possible. The cognitive psychology of writing confronts the practitioner with Otherness; experience can evidently be interpreted and valued in a variety of differing ways. The self-evident grip of naturalness is loosened. The practitioner is confronted with the unsettling potential of perspectivism, descriptions of in-service reality are open to interpretation, re-interpretation and doubt. The practitioner researcher writes up with his/her vocabulary; s/he conceptualizes experience relying on his/her perceptual schema (the organizing principles picked up through a life time) to categorize actions, infer intent and derive expectations. But an uncritical embrace of these presuppositions could lead to disaster:

> ".. an enormous amount of natural language is formulaic, automatic and rehears-ed, rather than propositional, creative or freely generated." (Fillmore, 1976)

If practitioners, without a commitment to a critical use of writing, merely confirm expectations and commonplace definitions, the resulting content will only lead to so many tautologies, self-fulfilling prophesies, and self-serving rationalizations. Practitioner research has to approach practice with an ability to recognize, formu-late, and work out judgments. Interpretation has to encourage a *critical* perspective. The researcher has to combine involvement and detachment – an insider's view with an outsider's perspective. A complex cognitive stance is necessary; concrete activity needs to be examined with a stereo-vision which juxtaposes practice and reflection. One has to live at the same time in two different cognitive worlds: (1) that of practice and (2) that of critical reflection. In the latter – second world of thought – the practitioner, via the examination of descriptions of practice, observes and analyses. This cognitive stance is characterized by the outsider's perspective. The effort of the teacher to analyze and explain practice on the basis of a written description, depends on the text being used as a mirror: to observe one's own work; to reflect on one's own strategies; to monitor on-going plans of action; and to manage change. The Insider's perspective provides the information which meets the needs of practitioner research. The practitioner compares what has happened in (a series of) interaction(s) to the criterion set in the external position. Thus, on the content level, what we call practitioner research, is a situation wherein a practition-er examines critically (the external viewpoint) an aspect of professional behaviour (the internal perspective). How open the practitioner will be for the outsider's critical perspective, determines the quality of the research. The critical perspective is grounded in the otherness that the practitioner achieves in writing-up events. This form of otherness is developed in contact with another person, namely with the facilitator.

I will further examine the dynamics of this crucial relationship in the next section. Thus, while the process of writing stimulates the development of distance to events, writing is not of itself synonymous with effective practitioner research.

Interactive principles

The observations which form the basis for practitioner research will only be illuminative if the teacher has a critical strategy which transforms daily reality into new insights. Entitlement and the cognitive skills are means of achieving this goal. The practitioner has to supplement normal perspectives on practice with a critical way of standing back from events. The quality of the distance taken from immediate practice is crucial; it determines if practitioner research will be misused to avoid critical experience or properly used to pursue it.

To summarize what has been said about the practitioner/facilitator relationship: the practitioner can only articulate his/her professional experience:

(1) thanks to an entitlement gained from the facilitator and

(2) with a cognitive stance which often needs facilitator encouragement.

In entitlement and via the cognitive skills, the teacher parts company with normal self-evident ways of looking at things. Practice is perceived to be worth researching and worth being examined from different perspectives. The facilitator has served as a catalyst, generating a critical perspective on practice. Recast in a simple formula:

$$\underset{\text{Entitlement + Cognitive skills}}{\overset{\text{(B)} \qquad \text{(C)}}{}} \; < \; \frac{\overset{\text{(B)} \qquad \text{(C)}}{\text{Entitlement + Cognitive skills}}}{\underset{\substack{\text{Principles of Interaction} \\ \text{Facilitator/Practitioner} \\ \text{relationship}}}{\text{(D)}}}$$

The combined effect of (B) entitlement and (C) the cognitive skills of in-practice investigation, add up to less than a successful facilitator/practitioner interaction. Entitlement (B) and the Cognitive Skills (C) are important instrumental tools, but no more than that. They form the content level of the facilitation, but the quality of the practitioner/facilitator interaction determines the process level. Clearly: practitioner research, is not doing research alone. Practitioner research cannot be done by oneself. This sounds self-contradictory. After all, practitioner research does entail the observing and studying of one's *own* actions. In effect the practitioner does field work on his/her own professional practice.[1] Even though practitioner research is a learning situation wherein one tries to assess one's own actions and activities, it remains socially, linguistically and structurally dependent upon the way practitioner activity is re-constituted in the interaction with the facilitator. What sort of practitioner/facilitator relationship is needed in practitioner research? To shed some light on this issue I will distinguish between three sorts of interact: (a) loose coupling, (b) single interact and (c) double-interact.[2]

In *loose coupling* we are confronted with a relationship of seriality: the sum of the whole is experientially less than the sum of the parts. In Non-Entitlement there is seriality; individual experience is richer than is shared experience. The non-involvement between individuals leads to doing ordinary; a mutual lack of interest destroys the very possibility of communication. When the Other/Practitioner relationship – between the social scientist and teacher – is loosely coupled there is little or no dialogue. The interaction is lukewarm and is most often characterized by the pattern: expert action meets with practitioner indifference. The facilitator degenerates into his/her professional monologue; the practitioner turns inward, isolated by a feeling of being excluded from important matters. The facilitator has defined in-practice experience as peripheral or insubstantial to expert social science knowledge. The social scientist assumes that practitioners are incapable of adequately making their own professional judgments or decisions.

In structures of *single interacts* one person acts, another reacts. The one initiates, the other responds. For instance, a researcher gives a practitioner an assignment such as: Observe gender-linked behaviours during work. When practitioner problem solving is based on facilitator competence (in a discipline or technique) there is a situation of single-interact.

Interaction is characterized by *double interact* when both interlocutors explicitly demonstrate insight into the viewpoint of the other. The definition of the double interact hinges on the relationship. The practitioner-facilitator double interact is characterized by interlocutors who try to come to terms with each other's way of looking at circumstance. When a practitioner and facilitator genuinely interact, the mutual recognition of each other's point of view is characteristic to the inter-action. Rational discussion often does not include any such insight into the other's outlook; it is dominated by (single interact) argumentation. The central premise to facilitating the double interact is not an individually held conviction in the rational truth of one's own stand-point, but the shared discovery of common understanding. Dialogue is grounded in a mutual awareness and respect of how the other person looks at (in-practice) reality. The communicative problem with social science *truth* is that (most often) it doesn't convince. People are not actually prepared to act on the outcomes of research, I submit, because they experience them as single interacts. (Armstrong, 1982) Only when one experiences agreement with a point of view (double interact), does one act on it. High quality practitioner research depends on being able to investigate in-service reality in a dialogue of differing, but genuinely experienced perspectives.

In the initial phase to practitioner research it is important to identify a felt information need. The teacher identifies a question where s/he has a direct personal interest in the answer. In the facilitator-practitioner relationship of double interact, a dialogue occurs where responses are sought to genuinely felt problems. This relationship goes against the grain of social conformity. Only problems where we do not know the solution (often we do not even know *if* there is a solution) lead to a dialogue. For instance, what are called in Dutch *Zwarte scholen* (*black schools*, i.e. schools attended by an overwhelming majority of immigrant and/or minority pupils) are eminently discussable because issues of integration/segregation, teacher motivation/demotivation, school success/school failure, order/disorder, involvement/disengagement are all posed without there being any clear answers or boundaries. In the logic of single interact facilitation, centring on expert opinions, problems are avoided; the social scientist does not share a problematic sense of an in-service context with the practitioner. In double interact facilitation, in-service reality is seen as open ended; there are no right answers. The teacher as researcher pursues context bound understanding, insight, action. The facilitator's role is different from the practitioner's; the practitioner wants to think through the particular needs of his/her circumstance, the facilitator represents the multiplicity of possible viewpoints and displays the indefinite character of practice. The practitioner needs a relationship of double interact with a facilitator to be free to raise questions, doubt practice, speculate about change. Double interacts are enabling. Rendered in an aphorism: behind practitioner research there is dialogue; in dialogue there is experimentation with many points of view.

Facilitation provides the prototype of seeing circumstance from a variety of perspectives. Obviously, the standards of interaction set during the facilitation are not solely determined by the facilitator. The double interact is based upon a mutual recognition of communication. Each party:

(1) understands what the other communicates and

(2) is aware that this understanding is present.

But if we try to describe practitioner research, we demand: What does a relationship of double interact look like? How do you know in a specific context whether there is a dialogue? How does one know if understanding is mutual? How can one see if communication really takes place? My reply is to adopt a negative definition of the facilitation process. I cannot define the behavioural pre-requisites to achieving double interact, but I can describe what one must *not* do. Facilitation grounded in double interacts can *not* be standardized. Inflexible standards would contradict the principle of open communication; they would compromise the conducting of context bound dialogue. In double interact each situation and person has to be understood on his/her own terms. The social scientist who is committed to practitioner research, is an inveterate opponent to formalism. S/he resists the tendency to divorce methods from context. *Not* an absolutely logical structure of ideas, but the development of practical maturity is the goal. *Not* standardized measurement but improved practice is the sought for. The facilitator does *not* assume that human experience is simple-minded and doctrinaire, but that it outruns rational concepts. One is *not* pursuing intellectual neatness but the variety and complexity of particulars. Questions are considered *not* in terms of generalizations but on the basis of the actual incongruities within which a coherent centre of intent and purpose is (often) recognizable. Critical judgments are directed by participants beliefs and *not* by imposed truths. The research is *not* guided by general standards of practice, but is concrete in its pursuit of circumstantial response. The facilitator values the in-practice circumstance for its own sake, and *not* because it corresponds to a prescribed model. The critical role is *not* separable from the creative one. The practitioner/facilitator interaction is *not* allowed to deteriorate into the dualism(s) of practice versus theory, activity versus criticism, description versus analysis. The need for critical research standards is *not* an appropriate basis for the division of labour. One must *not* polarize the relationship practitioner/social scientist along the lines: the former provides the experience, the latter the criteria for judgment. To do so makes dialogue impossible and destroys the very rigour which is sought for – the practitioner/facilitator relationship is *not* one of contraries but of complementaries. The facilitator and the practitioner keep the multiplicity of potential approaches alive in the research process. The research entails juxtaposing educational values – which are moral, aesthetic and social – with practice. There is no reason to assume that the values should be defined by the facilitator, nor to assume that the facilitator should blindly accept the practitioner's point of view. In a relationship of double interacts, values are negotiated; they are chosen in dialogue.

Introducing practitioner research in the Netherlands

The problem of transferability can now be explored with use of the conceptual model of practitioner research. Can practitioner research as developed by Nias, Day, Handal and Bell be introduced effectively in a foreign context, specifically in Holland? The distinction between two operational levels: the content of the relationship (Entitlement and Cognition of Practice) and its process (Double Interact versus Single Interact/Loose Coupling) has been emphasized. In the analysis of transferability the distinction between these two levels will play a prominent role. When we recast the conceptual model in a schema which instead of showing it as a system reveals the contraries involved, Figure 2 results.

Feeling (entitlement) is opposed here to thinking (cognitive skills) and dialogue (double interact) to monologue (loose coupling & single interact). The four terms define four quadrants, each characterized by a particular activity. All these activities are to be found in Dutch In-Service Training and/or Staff Development programmes:

- Work with in-service students has been directed towards Entitlement in a relationship of Double Interact which has focused on the Quality of Communication between the practitioner and facilitator, as well as between the

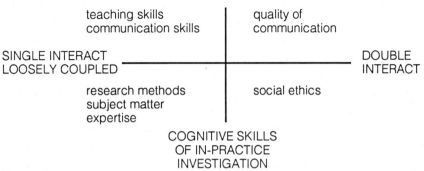

ENTITLEMENT

teaching skills   quality of
communication skills   communication

SINGLE INTERACT _____ DOUBLE
LOOSELY COUPLED   INTERACT

research methods   social ethics
subject matter
expertise

COGNITIVE SKILLS
OF IN-PRACTICE
INVESTIGATION

Figure 2

practitioner and his/her field. But the cognitive skills of in-practice investigation have all too often been delegated to the facilitator, who may even take such tasks over for her/his very own: i.e. the facilitator writes up the research results for the practitioner.

- Some facilitators have emphasized the development of the Cognitive Skills of In-Practice Investigation within a practitioner/instructor relationship of Double Interact. Hereby the Social Ethics of schooling / learning / training have become a crucial point of concern. The quality to the person-person and/or group-group interaction was examined. Reflection on the theory-practice relationship has resulted.

- Often there has been a relationship of Single Interact or Loose Coupling between instructors/facilitators and practitioners; an Imparting of Teaching / Communication Skills, or instruction in Research Techniques and Subject Matter Expertise has taken place. The assumption is: when practitioners master the basal techniques of teaching and/or in-practice research, they will be ready and able to improve their own practice. Facilitation offers guide-lines. Once basic skills are mastered, the facilitator continues to offer tips to improve and ensure utilization. For the practitioner the activity is guided by rules set forth by the facilitator; most often this leads to practitioner resistance and/or passivity! At best practitioners *do* the research required of them.

Though the Dutch listener can say in all honesty: I've heard it all already; what's new here?, the introduction of practitioner research, congruent with Les Bell's, Chris Day's, Gunnar Handal's and Jennifer Nias's ideas would represent a radical break in Dutch pedagogic practice. This sort of practitioner research would be found, in the schema above, equidistant between Entitlement and Cognitive Skills of In-Practice Investigation; and high in Double Interact. Practitioners who openly examine their own criteria of judgment and observe their own actions to check their social effectiveness, appropriateness and consistency, are engaged in this type of activity. Virtually no practitioner research, in this sense, has been done in Holland. The presence of the component parts (Figure Two) does *not* imply the presence of the whole (i.e. of the system as shown in Figure One)! The crucial factor is to be found in the relationship between the pedagogue (social scientist) and the practitioner (teacher).

I now want to examine one of the presuppositions to the relationship between the two stakeholders, the teacher and the pedagogue, namely their social positions. It is hard to think of an instance in which the field of pedagogics has been changed solely for the sake of improving the teacher/pedagogue relationship, and thereby education. Problems of research effectiveness and/or the facilitation of teacher improvement are never the *only* interests promoted. Pedagogic change typically occurs for nonpedagogic ends: stakeholder (elite) positions play a central role. The paradigm shift which took place in pedagogics in Holland during the early seventies promoted the position of a (mostly social democratic) technocratic elite at the cost of the old (mostly Christian Democrat) personalist one. Current efforts to create a buyers market for In-Service Training and/or Staff Development promotes the position of (mostly liberal) managers to the detriment of the (mostly functionalist) institutional providers of training/staff development. At issue in the future of practitioner research is the creation of a new elite and/or the maintenance of an old one. The currently dominant pedagogic elite asserts that the unprecedented knowledge and wealth of the modern society is based on a complex division of labour. Science and formal organization foster the rational determination of social ends and means. Relations of community, characterized by strong ties to others, have been replaced by highly differentiated role behaviour (expertness) in order to achieve effectiveness via rationality. Practitioner research represents an unwanted return to a pre-scientific idealization of the simple, intimate community. The opposing new elite emphasizes the dynamic facet of society. Tensions between differing personalities, groups, generations can only be productive if acknowledged, studied, and openly dealt with. Social and technological development not only cannot, but should not, be controlled by an expert elite. There is no meta-level truth superior to direct experiential involvement. The old elite wants to (continue to) organize education along hierarchical bureaucratic lines; the new elite champions a flat, flexible management model. The present Dutch situation is paradoxical: the quality of schooling is quite good but the educational management is notoriously slow and ineffective (see Van der Wolf & Ramaekers, in this volume). The current elite though managerially ineffective can defend its position: Why should we change if the educational system is delivering the goods? A new Practitioner Research elite could answer: The rich tacit knowledge of the practitioners makes the educational system effective; the static produced by the pedagogic elite is at best irrelevant and at worst dangerous. In practitioner research the pedagogue nurtures practitioner tacit knowledge and insight. The pedagogue helps the practitioner to hold a mirror up to practice. A privileged tool herein is the exemplary use of one's powers of description. Such a pedagogue resembles more the generation of Langeveld and Buytendijk (mid 1940s to mid 1960's) than that of Van Kemenade and Imelman (1970s and 1980s).[3] A descriptive pedagogics is preferred to a policy driven *dirigist* one. Practitioner research attempts in fact to redefine the task of the pedagogic elite.

Who could instigate practitioner research (as defined above) for Dutch teachers and *how?* Re-defined and targeted: How can the language behaviour of Dutch teachers be changed so that they would write, evaluate, criticize, and act upon their own descriptions of practice? Who has, or could develop, a mandate to initiate a deliberate policy of in-service training and staff development whereby the practitioner researcher resources of the teaching community would be pur posefully organized and developed? We are neither looking for intellectual persuasion (for instance, as attempted in this book), nor for support from a practitioner constituency (for instance, as attempted by CARN)[4], but for an organized attempt to foster practitioner research via in-service training and staff development.

Under what conditions and through what policy-making process could practitioner research become important in Holland? For two reasons one cannot simply follow a foreign (British) model.

Firstly, the teacher-as-researcher movement in the UK dates from twenty years ago. Its beginnings and development took place in a very different cultural/political/social circumstance than that of today. Intellectual attitudes were different: then *alienation* was in the forefront of the intelligentsia's attention, now *Postmodernism* is au courant. Practitioner Research reflects the philosophical spirit of the fifties and sixties. The pursuit of the other: as repression or liberation, as dehumanizing technocracy or humanizing unity, as deadening or enabling, are all typical of the existential influence. The idea that practitioners can potentially find an authentic relationship with a facilitator is radically optimistic. A more contemporary voice: "Philosophy and psychology died at the same moment as the other, and the desire for the other, died. Only the empty sign of their content shines out now .." (Baudrillard, 1990) The simulacrum is characteristic of current thought: the individual may pursue the appearance of relationship, but s/he will never find it. The pursuit of the double – the assumption that one can find the same humanity in the other as one finds in oneself – is typical of existentialism. Current thinking is more apt to assert that the pursuit of the double does *not* lead to dialogue (double interact), but merely to narcissistic illusion. Instead of discovering shared humanity the subject indulges in egocentric projection, i.e. in generating a simulacrum (fantasy/image) of the other which is a mirror image of the desires, fears, needs, of the consciousness producing the simulacrum. The everyday, unexamined uncritical assumptions of reality, cannot be challenged by engagement with a double (entitlement, cognitive skills, double interact) as Action Research would wish; consciousness itself is threatened by the sheer idiocy of circumstance. Classroom education maintains the discourse of the simulacrum; it tells truths, instructs facts, demands respect for rules. Teachers pretend that essentialism has been a success: We know what nature, society, history are really all about. Postmodernism challenges the modernist (simulacrum) myth: there is no privileged access to a truth which is lying somewhere behind appearance. The desperate attempt to snatch meaning out of practice is understandable enough, but what can it achieve? The old hope, that man can somehow get the better of alienation, is gone. What Postmodernists doubt in Practitioner Research is not the value of talking to one another, but that this talking leads to something that ought to be called research. The *discursive* (analyzed, reasoned) text of research is opposed to *a cursive* (flowing, impromptu) form of writing. Postmodernism suffers from the crushing ambiguity towards *the other* characteristic of its most important precursor: Nietzsche. An intense desire for mutual understanding is coupled to an almost total despair of man's ability to be honest to him/herself and/or to others. The simulacrum – the comfortable illusion of purpose, truth, reason, order – overwhelms experiential reality, making genuine interaction impossible. The simulacrum presents us with an ultravisible, ultrareal, transparent world of effectivity; Postmodernism tries to juxtapose an uncertain, indefinite, indescribable world of interacts, to the world of mindless effect and technological glitter. In so far as persons *converse* in Practitioner Research it remains utterly contemporary; in so far as an ambition for educational progress or social truth lives on in it, it is a child of the simulacrum of the fifties and sixties. For Practitioner Research a significant postscript to having begun in the Britain of the 50's and 60's is that (at least) some institutional support (University of East Anglia / Cambridge Institute of Euucation) was realizable; I assume because the simulacrum reaffirmed the progressive/social democratic assumptions that were then current.

Secondly, the social/political context was, and is, very different in Britain as compared to Holland. In the Britain of today state supported schooling is widely perceived to NOT deliver the goods. The difference with Holland is not one of comparative educational performance (which we know very little about) but of political sensibility (i.e. of the position of the political elite). Thus practitioner research in Holland cannot ride a wave of anti-socialist government sentiment[5]. The Dutch society/economy resembles more the German (to which it is intimately linked) than the British. Its values are more production oriented than service directed. The process of radical restructuring wherein Britain halved its industrial economy (1980-90) has barely started in Holland (with the crisis in Philips). In the Netherlands the shift from production values (engineering and technique predominate) to market values (service and flexibility stand central) is probably just beginning. The educational *engineer* focuses on achieving pre-set quantified results; educational flexibility tries to generate new forms of learning. The ideals (self-admittedly inachievable) of the dominant pedagogic elite are planned change and expert-control. How would the acknowledgement that education is messy, specific and uncontrollable, be beneficial? As long as educational power can be patterned hierarchically, pedagogic elites can (seem to) act unilaterally and government can (apparently) act directly on school policy; why change? Of course real influence on in-practice reality is scant; genuine acceptance of expert opinion is minimal. The authority of the pedagogic elite is absent. It cannot enforce its assertions; there are virtually no punishments for non-compliance. The real authority of academic pedagogues amongst teachers is notoriously weak. Negative incentives (If you do not do what we want, we will not give you *x* amount of money) often seem to be the only operative power. Teacher response is grudging and bitter. But no counter-elite has mustered support. The legitimacy of the ruling elite may be weak, but no alternative has mobilized teacher enthusiasm[6]. To summarize: the bond between the pedagogic elite and teachers is characterized by (very) loose coupling, but no alternative form of interact (counter-elite) has effectively asserted itself. Thus which social/political conditions and resulting policy initiatives, can be realistically anticipated that would permit practitioner research to gain a substantial influence?

A **first scenario**: the current growth in economic competitiveness with its emphasis on efficiency and individual competency has created a growth market for work-related training. Private training and consulting organizations have profited; the pedagogic elite (working in the state subsidized sector) has occupied a minimal, peripheral position. The pedagogic professionals have failed to develop new products, offer innovative services or find a new proactive niche for themselves. The people who are supposed to be experts in facilitating professional growth, curriculum development, evaluation techniques, didactic innovation, the applications of new technologies to learning, and educational research have been ineffective. The school teachers have taught school more or less as if the new market for in-service training did not exist; the pedagogues have not reacted to the potential new market(s). In the sectors of organizational consulting and commercial training a counterelite has developed. This counterelite is narrowly commercial in its behaviour, pedagogically conservative in its conceptualization of learning, and focusses in its attitude to learning materials on short term results.The presentation of programmes is often done with more care than is the determination of content; the result of *happiness sheets* often is more important than is learning; the instant delivery of skills prevails often over significant personal development. The market niche for high quality in-service training is largely open. But the pedagogic elite has long been accustomed to a sellers market wherein in-service training has served as a cash cow. Guaranteed income from government, coupled to a minimum of competition, did not put a premium on high quality innovative programming. Because it has never had to work efficiently (client and service directed, keeping within a budget) or entrepreneurially, the pedagogic elite is ill-prepared to enter the new in-service training market. The pedagogic elite has preferred to accept redundancies than to change its ways. A more proactive strategy could lead pedagogics into a new market where practitioner research would be very valuable. But the prerequisite change in work culture would be significant. A restructuring of the professional self-image would be necessary; the traditional position which assumes a social hierarchy of labour based on an intellectual hierarchy of knowledge, would have to be abandoned for one of social partnership (with teachers) based on an experiential/process concept of knowledge. The normal resistance to change will work against the implementation of any such innovation; furthermore, the realization by the pedagogic elite that it might not retain its privileges makes the alternative unattractive to it. Thus the stakeholder's position of the pedagogic elite is paradoxical: practitioner research threatens established positions while it provides growth opportunities. Even though old positions have been (partially) eroded by government budget cuts, the pedagogic elite has not tried to re-define its activities. While the logic for getting into the new practitioner research market is there, the resistance to any such adventure is (for the moment) equally strong.

Put in terms of the conceptual model: the threat to academic identity and to self-status of the double interact dissuades the pedagogic elite from entering into practitioner research, even though the benefit in entitlement (having something meaningful to say) is evident.

A **second scenario**: the Ministry of Education, probably in an effort to save money, chooses to devolve authority over in-service training and staff development to the school. For instance, secondment (now unknown in Holland) could be introduced as a way of employing more teachers while lowering the overall budget (teachers cost less than do school trainers and advisers). In theory devolution gives the school the chance to make choices concerning its own in-service training and staff development. The sellers market (trainers and advisers do pretty much what they want) is replaced by a buyers market (the school gets what it demands). But for practitioner research there is the danger that the schools will go for the *quick fix*, i.e. favour training which promises maximum results with a minimum of effort. Furthermore just as long as there are few pay incentives for Dutch teachers to perform better, there may not be sufficient material stimuli to encourage teachers to choose the more challenging and demanding path. Though practitioner research potentially offers an ideal fit between practitioner and pedagogue, it demands hard work of both. Neither party may be motivated to engage itself so thoroughly. A factor mitigating against a teacher-pedagogue *do-nothing pact* is that those schools which are perceived to be qualitatively superior are flourishing, and those perceived to be weak are loosing pupils. There is a good chance that up-market, middle class schools will go in for practitioner research; and that down-market inner city, ghetto schools will not. Furthermore the high quality, rich neighbourhood schools are more often part of small school districts with few administrators; the less privileged schools are often part of a large school district with a large bureaucracy. The logic of administration will lead the former to let their principals choose which in-service training and staff development is wanted, and the latter to let their administrators do so. In the former case the schools will actively enter the new market as buyers and search out the best offerings; in the latter case the bureaucracies will stick to their established contacts and re-use existing programmes. The difference between mediocre schools and privileged ones will thus be increased. I would expect that a fairly limited number of relatively high quality schools would choose to make the depth investment in their human resources which practitioner research demands. In situations of crisis management – low achieving pupils, rapid staff turnover – practitioner research probably doesn't make much sense. Since the number of pedagogues who are either qualified or motivated to work on practitioner research is limited, this scenario is tenable on the supply as well as demand sides. In terms of the conceptual model, only in *some* schools will the teachers be interested and encouraged to develop their cognitive skills. The sense of professional entitlement (*My work is important*) which encourages teachers to improve their practitioner reflective skills will be related to the academic quality of the school. The cognitively better schools will get still better, and the weaker schools will become relatively even weaker. The double interact will be a form of privileged teacher/ pedagogue contact, open only to a practitioner elite.

A **third scenario**: an institution of higher education decides to champion practitioner research as a way of expressing its particularity. A prerequisite to such a strategy succeeding is that a sufficiently experienced group of practitioner researchers could be brought together to develop and run the programme. To be effective such a team would have to be able to put on appropriate degree granting courses such as M.Ed's (Masters of Education) or M.O.B.'s/H.K.P. degrees (the Dutch professional MA level degree in Education). Such an initiative would be launching itself on an uncharted course of academic deviance. The denunciations that *There is no proof of effectiveness* and that *The programme is unscientific* could come fast and thick. If the programme was started as a Dutch - British partnership (such as the MBS cooperation with Twente University); or as a British institution in Holland (such as Bradford University's Utrecht Management School) the attack on the programme's legitimacy would be muted. Up to now practitioner research in Holland has had a British connection: the conference which preceded this book included several British speakers and was first proposed on a British Rail train between Nottingham and London[7]; the CPS Teacher Action

Research Conference was a CARN related initiative and included John Elliott as speaker (Elliott, 1987); the Nutsseminarium teacher-as-researcher projects were supported by Gordon Bell's EC research funds (Letiche, 1985); and a Self-Evaluation Conference was also funded by Bell's project. (Letiche, 1988b) It is not clear that an independent centre for practitioner research is possible in Holland: would there be enough expertise, interest and commitment? Further-more, would such a Centre for Practitioner Research be able to do original crea-tive work? A merely imitative programme probably could not survive. In terms of the conceptual model, this third scenario elegantly solves the entitlement issue by making use of borrowed legitimacy. But it is not certain that one can bundle enough cognitive and process skills in a single (new) centre to be effective.

Conclusion

The first scenario was problematic because there seemed to be no reason for the current pedagogic elite to spontaneously commit itself to striving for a relation-ship of double interact with practitioners. The second scenario was uncertain because the investment in developing new cognitive skills demanded of practi-tioner researchers seemed unlikely to be made by teachers from any but the best of schools. The third scenario seems to be the most attractive because it (in part) solves the problem of legitimacy, i.e. of its own entitlement, without expending lots of valuable resources on that parameter. This would leave a prospective Centre for Practitioner Research free to engage all its energy in organizing in-service projects. If such a Centre has to battle both to achieve its own entitlement and to be cognitively effective, it would probably be stretched too thin to survive. The battle of entitlement threatens to force any initiative back into ordinary science (i.e. into doing ordinary). But there is no guarantee that entitlement, appropriate research (cognitive) skills, and the commitment to working in double interact can all be marshalled by one staff in one place. Practitioner research remains a difficult juggling act wherein three different balls have to be kept in the air at once. We know from abroad that it can be done, but have yet to prove our ability to follow suit. While elements could be mixed from the three scenarios, the third one seems at present the most promising.

Notes

1. "This approach to social investigation has traditionally been asociated with social anthropologists, whose 'field' consisted of a small-scale society where it was possile to do 'research' by living and working among the people. ...The

main instrument of ... investigation is the researcher, who has to ... live among the people and participate in their activities over relatively long periods of time in order to acquire a detailed understanding of the situation under study."

See Burgess, Robert (1982), *Field Research: a Sourcebook and Field Manual.* London:.George Allen & Unwin

2. The terms come from the organizational psychologies of Karl Weick (1979) and Henk van Dongen (in Willem de Laat, 1985).

3. Characteristic for the phenomenologist Buytendijk:

   F.J.J. Buytendijk (1948), *Algemene Theorie de Menselijke Houding en Beweging.* Utrecht, Het Spectrum (translated in German 1956, French 1957).

   Characteristic for the Personalist Langeveld:

   M.J. Langeveld (1944), *Beknopte Theoretische Paedagogiek.* Groningen: Wolters (other books published in German in the '60s).

   Characteristic of the Critical Rationalist Imelman:

   J.D. Imelman (1977), *Inleiding in de Pedagogiek* Groningen: Wolters-Noordhoff.

   Characteristic for the Sociologist of Education Van Kemenade:

   J. van Kemenade (1986), *Onderwijs bestel en beleid* Groningen: Wolters-Noordhoff.

4. Classroom Action Research Network (Cambridge UK) which organized with the CPS (Christelijk Pedagogisch Studiecentrum) a practitioners conference on the teacher-as-researcher. Appropriately enough the representative of the Dutch Ministry or Education dismissed the problem of a gap between teachers and academics as irrelevant to the Dutch context!

5. In fact, the present Minister of education is a socialist.

6. Statements based on my own and my research assistants observations; there has not as yet been a significant amount of rigorous research into these issues.

7. Kees van de Wolf and I were returning from the ISATT Conference in Nottingham.

❖❖❖ III ❖❖❖

IN-SERVICE TRAINING AND STAFF-DEVELOPMENT IN THE NETHERLANDS

Chapter 6

EDUCATIONAL POLICY FOR SCHOOL DEVELOPMENT

Fons van Wieringen, University of Amsterdam

Institutions for assisting schools

Individual pupils with problems in school have been assisted since the start of this century by agencies working in the medical and/or psychological areas. Services ranging from dentistry to tests for career choice have been available to pupils. In the course of this century these services have gradually been expanded to include a broad range of help for individuals with social and/or cognitive problems; problems which were at least partially related to school performance. In addition, the schools themselves have been targeted for help from the same institutions which assist pupils. In the last three decades a growing number of professionally staffed institutions have taken on the objective of offering assistance and support to schools and/or of changing and improving schools.

In the Netherlands the institutions at the regional and the national level include, for example: regional centres for helping schools and pupils; national institutes for curriculum and test development; national centres for consultancy, research and documentation. These institutions are state subsidized and for the most part governed by a board of governors consisting of representatives of different stakeholders in the educational system. As a whole, these institutions can be characterized as: state dependent for their budget and governed semi-autonomously by a coalition of different stakeholders. Internally there is a dual order to the organization of the institutions: on one hand they have a governing board in which political and religious interests are represented, and on the other their own professionals play a crucial role in their activity. In those institutions where the professional (technical) core and/or services are clearly developed, for example in the Institute for Test Development, the governing board at the institutional level generally does not do any harm to the necessary professional orientation. On the other hand, in institutions where the professional (technical) level is less clearly developed, for example centres for general school support, the crystalization of professional standards is a more difficult process. The total system of institutions for supporting schools can, therefore, be seen dualistically, either as oriented towards the political (stakeholder) process in their boards, or as oriented towards their own professional standards. Clients are stakeholders in the political or professional process but have a very limited influence. As we shall see later, this shortcoming is at the moment a focus of reform. The insufficient orientation towards clients is also reflected in the imperfect coordination between the different institutions in their interaction with schools. The support offered is not clearly coordinated or geared to the specific needs of schools.

I note that the Institutes for Pre- and In-Service Teacher Training are not included in the system of school support institutions. They have been placed in a different institutional category, i.e. that of higher education. Nevertheless, they are characterized by the same factors: state financing, semi-autonomous boards of governors, an internal organizational model which is professionally oriented.

The funding agencies

Such a support system with two sub-systems – a teacher training sub-system and a specialized support sub-system – could only come into existence if the state funding system and corresponding system of schools made this possible. As far as the state is concerned: the financial policy was very generous in the 60's and 70's (it was not yet constrained by budget restrictions); subsidizing went directly to the institutions which offered professional services, i.e. the supply side was subsidized; the Ministry of Education saw the support institutions to a significant degree as instruments for executing the aims of national educational policy. The primary and secondary school system, in its own way, encouraged the creation of the support system just sketched. The systems of schools can be said to consist of:
- moderate to small sized schools, i.e. too small to be able to have specialized support functions within the school; schools have no budgetary means to buy in external services. The schools are to a large degree dependent on the services offered to them by the institutions.
- schools which are not stimulated by any budgetary mechanism to make articulated demands for specific services which they really need.
- schools which even if they could have their own budget to buy external expertise, would be very little motivated to take the initiative. The impetus for buyers-behavior is lacking because almost all aspects of the school operation are highly regulated through national contracts between the teacher unions, the national associations of school boards and the government. As a consequence,

schools traditionally have had little room for policies of their own. Policy making by schools was discouraged by the detailed prescriptions sent to schools, at regular intervals, from the national level.

Since the early 1980's some of the afore mentioned has changed. Although one can analyze the general direction of change, and I will attempt just that here, there is of course only a general re-orientation which is not yet realized in all its details. For some areas, the change from input regulation to strict output policy is still being debated in terms of the main lines of future policy. Essentially, the economic crisis of the welfare state gave rise to a process of questioning the structure and functioning of the dual system of support. Were schools better-off with such a dual support system? What have been the effects of the services delivered? Several research projects were created to try to gauge the effectiveness of the system. As one can imagine, the research met with differing degrees of success. Thus, the first step towards questioning and improving the support system was to carry out several research projects. The second step was to design alternative principles for organizing the support system. Simply said, it has been decided that the system should be more consumer-oriented, client-directed and financed directly by the school. Finally, budget cutting has taken advantage of the decision that the dual system had not been adequately effective.

Deregulation and responsibility for budgets

In the Netherlands, responsibility for in-service training was allocated to the Colleges of Education in 1976. Financial means for the in-service training of teachers were provided by the central government. Decisions about the use of the money slated for in-service training was in part a responsibility of the government, after consultation with national school board associations and the unions; and in part a responsibility of the Colleges of Education. New policy in the financing of in-service training amounts to a shrinking of government funding which used to cover 50% of the budget. This percentage is being reduced and the funds remaining will be used for specific in-service training goals meeting national priorities such as multi-cultural education. The Colleges of Education are gradually becoming less influential as suppliers, in comparison to the demanders of training. In a first stage, the colleges were expected to offer courses according to their own vision of school needs. In a second stage, course offerings were expected to be based on requests from the schools, i.e. from teachers. The budget for in-service training is being transferred to the primary and secondary schools in such a way that the schools gain an ear marked budget for buying in-service training either from the Colleges of Education or from other suppliers from within or from outside the educational sector. Government legitimation for such a change in subsidizing policy is to be found, in general, in a re-orientation wherein central policy and regulations are, up to a certain degree, withdrawn; and in specific, in the assertion that schools should be more autonomous.

Up to now educational policy in the Netherlands is not only centralized but also highly detailed and specified in its numerous regulations. The balance of power between the different social-religious groups, and the form of accommodation they have found in the one nation-state, has resulted in a legalistic policy system where much energy is spent in specifying the general rules, the rules for specific situations, the rules for exceptions to the general rules and/or exceptions to the rules for specific situations, the general rules for allowing exceptions, the rules for exceptions to the rules governing exceptions, etc, etc., etc. This system of regulations was stimulated by an attempt in the '60's and '70's to initiate an active educational policy; the net effect of which was an added stimulus to the rule making mania of the system.

Budgetary problems and an ideological re-orientation from planning to market forces, has challenged the rule-making system. In consequence, a policy of de-regulation for the educational sector has been initiated. The starting point for this policy shift has been higher education, including the Colleges of Education (the teacher training faculties of the Polytechnics). Higher education has traditionally been the educational sector, in comparison to primary and secondary education, governed the least by central regulations. The first area for deregulation was financial. Institutions of higher education are now financed by a system of lump sum grants and no longer by a detailed system of declarations. This gives the universities and colleges much more freedom in deciding budgetary priorities. Having now been implemented in higher education, this system of lump sum funding is presently being introduced in primary an secondary education. As a result, the schools will have more financial options and possibilities to use their means to meet their own school priorities.

Policy making on the school level

One pole of the deregulation operation is that of the government, the other is that of the school. Deregulation is not only a matter of central government doing less or doing things differently, it is also a matter of stimulating and enabling schools to set their own priorities. This side of the operation is generally referred to as the growth in autonomy and policy making capacity of schools. This growth is encouraged by various means, the most important of which are:
- enlarging the average size of educational institutions and school boards. This policy originated in the higher education sector; the number of Colleges of Higher Education was reduced from about 400 to 80 in a couple of years. This

process of amalgamation and concentration is now also being carried out in Colleges for Further Education and Community Colleges. The same trend is to be found in secondary and primary education. However, the institutional size of schools can only be enhanced to a limited degree. Efforts, however, are being made to enlarge the number of schools governed by the same board. Lump sum funding is then to be granted by one board to run five to eight (primary) schools.

– the second instrument used to enlarge the policy making capacity of schools is to stimulate the development of the internal capacity of the schools in matters of curriculum development, staff differentation and school management. The curriculum is supposed to become more flexible by introducing a module-like work pattern, staff differentiation is expected to offer better opportunities for good teachers to develop their qualifications, and the training of school managers will create a body of professionals with the qualities needed to initiate and coordinate school-based decision making aimed at setting and implementing priorities in mission, strategy and operations.School strategies will need to be written down in school development plans in which general aims and missions are formulated. Sections of such a plan should describe the school curriculum, its students, housing, current expenditures and personnel. As far as the personnel are concerned, the school strategy needs to deal with problems like recruiting new staff members, guidance of staff, reward policies, et cetera. Policy towards in-school and out-of-school, in-service training of individual teachers and teams of teachers should be included in the school strategy. By giving schools a budget of their own to meet their training costs schools are encouraged to integrate training into their general personnel policy.

Contents and methods of in-service training

It is in a context of larger institutions which are better equipped to set their own internal policies, that the budgets for external assistance and support are being transferred to the schools. To assess the possible effects of this transfer for the Colleges of Education and for schools, we must examine in-service training in detail. What are the contents of the in-service training? What methods are used? How does the `market' for training presently work?

The contents of in-service training concentrate on subject matter material such as arithmetic, science, reading, foreign languages, et cetera. Programmes focused on national priorities in educational policy such as information technology, cultural-ethnic groups, emancipation, form the only important exception to the subject matter focus. The relationship between the contents (subjects) chosen and the target group one has in mind (methods) reveals four options (Figure 1):

	Subjects	
Methods ↓	One specific subject	Boundary crossing between subjects
Geared at individual teachers	Qualification development	Qualification and teaching repertoire development
Geared at teams of teachers from one school	Department/ section development	Schooldevelopment

Figure 1

Four possible forms of in-service training are revealed. At this moment the first cell (subject matter qualification development) is especially popular and to a lesser degree the third one (department/section development). School development (fourth quadrant) is at present the variant least frequently made use of in in-service training, though such in-service training is obviously suited to stimulating the school's capacity for internal policy making. But will it be chosen (i.e. bought) by schools? What will be the mix of different subject/method combinations which will emerge from the policy-making process in the specific schools?

New actors, new relations

The present situation is contrasted with the new one in Figure 2.
In the new situation stakeholders will interrelate in a different way. Furthermore, there are two new stakeholders in the field: the schools as such are new actors, and other suppliers than the Colleges of Education are coming into the picture. As a result all actors will (have to) behave in different ways.

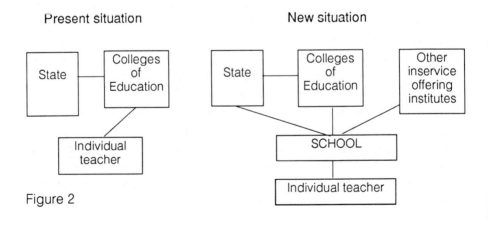

Figure 2

Van Wieringen ❖❖❖

The central government is changing its position from direct intervention to that of exerting influence at a distance. The Colleges of Education face two new actors. First of all, they will have to sell their services to schools in a market situation. The ability to listen carefully to the wishes and needs of schools will be needed. Furthermore, one will have to invest a lot of energy in fostering good working relations with a large number of individual schools if one is going to be successful. The other new actor confronting the Colleges of Education is the profit or non-profit organization which decides to offer in-service training. The competition between the traditional and new in-service training suppliers may well become quite uncomfortable for the colleges who are neither prepared nor very well equipped to defend their market.

The individual teacher will also act differently in the new situation. Formerly, s/he simply applied (or did not apply) to register for in-service courses at a college. His/her action had no financial implications for the school. In the new situation the individual wish for in-service training must be balanced with colleagues' and school needs. General staff needs and policy will be important in deciding who should follow which course. The individual need will have to compete for budgetary priority with school, department and sector needs, which have been formulated in (mini-)personnel plans.

From in-service training to human resource development

Schools will have a number of distinct policy variants to decide between when allotting their in-service training budgets. This can be best understood as a set of options (de Caluwé, Marx, and Petri, 1988):
— the budget can simply be equally divided between departments and teachers,
— the budget can be used according to a formal annual plan drafted for the school as a whole,
— the budget can be set as a part of a planning process including more than one year and a whole range of priorities,
— the budget can be incorporated in a broader framework of personnel policy or human resource development policy,
— the budget can be seen as a part of a human resource development strategy answering to the mission & strategy statements of the school, and linking human resource development with the current level of expenditures on housing, external relationships, public affairs, et cetera of the school.

One cannot, of course, be sure what choices schools are going to make. One can only hope that the in-service budget will be seen in relation to the other instruments of personnel policy. These instruments include recruiting, guidance, counselling, financial rewards, immaterial rewards, career patterning, task differentiation, et cetera. By transferring the in-service training budget to schools and, at the same time, giving the schools more options in other areas, one can provide for at least some of the conditions needed for creating an integrated human resource development policy in the school.

If the schools are open to change, then I expect that the external assistance and support offered to them will be reorganized. If both sides of the dual external support system, i.e. the in-service teacher training budget as well as the external support budget, are transferred to schools, a new pattern of differentiation in in-service training and the services offered should emerge. After all, the various aspects of professionalization beg for a more integrated approach. In-service training and the providing of expert advice/information via consultancy/organizational development can be provided in a much more client-oriented way, and coordinated so that staff learning is increased. Such an integrated offering of external assistance and support fits a climate where internal school policy embraces different aspects of human resources development. The coordination between different offerings and institutions may partly result from market forces in which the client, i.e. the school, has a central place. But probably something more is needed to strengthen coordination. Something like a broker may be needed to stimulate the processes of coordination. It will be very interesting to see which institutions try to become brokers for in-service training, staff development and school development.

Chapter 7

SOCIAL SCIENTISTS AS SORCERER'S APPRENTICES:
THE POLLUTED RELATIONS BETWEEN PRACTITIONERS AND EXPERTS

Maarten van den Dungen, University of Amsterdam

Introduction

The starting point for this discussion is the ambivalent attitude of teachers towards social science. This attitude can be easily observed. Sometimes it is stated openly, and sometimes it is expressed indirectly by ignoring given advice. The remark most often heard is that there is a wide gap between theory and every day reality. This appears, for example, in the fact that the ideas and suggestions put forward by "science" quite often cannot be realized, and on top of that are often not even found to be relevant. For that matter this does not just concern teachers. In other areas symptoms of an unsatisfactory and disrupted relationship between science and practice can also be found; this particularly applies to pedagogical care and welfare work. The consequences of these disrupted relationships are serious and far-reaching. On the one hand these are manifest in the conflicts between practitioners and scientific supervisors – quite often in one and the same educational or welfare organization. On the other hand we can observe deep dissatisfaction with existing refresher and continuing-education courses, which according to many do not achieve the objectives aimed for. Lastly – and not least importantly – such disturbances affect the working pleasure as well as the effectiveness of all parties involved, researchers as well the practitioners. It is not surprising then that in educational spheres the following statement is heard more and more often: "... schools themselves know best what kind of training is necessary for their specific circumstances". A further analysis of this area of tension – also described in this book by Nias as the relationship between *silencer* and *silenced* – is therefore badly needed. Our intention is twofold: firstly, we want to discover which factors play a role in the origin of these difficulties, and secondly we hope that this analysis will provide a basis for working out measures that contribute towards reducing the tension.

One of the most important factors contributing to the tension, we shall argue, is the distinction between knowledge acquired by means of scientific research as well as theoretical reflection, and insight gained through practical experience. In the course of time, as a result of this distinction science and practical activity have started to develop along separate roads. The difference extends a lot further than is often thought, and has a number of undesirable consequences. It has led, among other things, to a gap between education and training on the one hand, and practical experience on the other. This gap particularly makes itself felt in the social sector (as in education and social care). Its cause is twofold. On the one hand the object aimed at is not tangible and therefore there is little chance to pin it down when dealing with it. On the other hand there is (probably for the same reason) a strong tendency in education to concentrate mainly on the passing on of abstract (scientifically justifiable) theories and models. It is too often overlooked that in the practical situation a high level of knowledge acquisition also takes place.

I wish to concentrate, in the first instance, on the question *Whether and to what extent social science can indeed be characterized as a silencer.* Does science silence the practitioners who carry out the actual work? That is to say, does it – by its nature and way of acting – hamper their development? Or in other words, what factors adversely influence the relationship science / practice? I will focus attention on social science as a possible source of (intellectual or professional) repression. For the sake of balance, however, I will have to take into account that we are dealing with disfunctions within a system of relationships. Thus it would be dangerous to concentrate solely on (social) science as the possible source of conflict. We must widen our viewpoint. Initially I will give a brief description of science, as well as of practical experience. Thereafter I will discuss the relationship between science and practical experience; a relationship which is often referred to as technology. We will see that this concept leads to misunderstanding.

Science

Science as we know it today emerged (approximately) in the seventeenth century. At that time radical changes took place which gave (Western) society a very different appearance. The changes concerned the way reality was looked at (and also thus the way reality was dealt with). People became increasingly aware of the power of rationalism. Western man started to consider ideas as being more important than sensory perceptions. This led to a changed attitude towards the acquiring of knowledge. Logical reasoning and strict observation within the framework of logically built up questioning, was seen to be the appropriate way of acquiring reliable knowledge about nature. Experimentation is an approach which meets these requirements. Supposedly, only by experimenting can one find out how the world is really constructed. An approach was being developed which made it possible for the thinking theoretician and the experimenting engineer to confront each other.

The results of this revolution in thinking were far-reaching. If ideas are more important than experience in research, then one should be led as little as possible by sense perception. A predilection for external constructions ensues. Ideas, posited to stand outside the world of perception (i.e. theories leading to the formulation of research questions), were the starting point for research (i.e. serving as hypotheses to be empirically tested). Thus the researcher, distanced as much as possible from sense perception, decides the subject of, and methodology for, research. In result the knowledge acquired has a distant, abstract quality to it. It does not reflect (primarily) a unique phenomenon. On the contrary, by means of theory and testing, an overall insight into the collections of phenomena is aimed for. It is not the particular tree that matters but trees in general (or a specific kind of tree, under certain circumstances).

I do want to try to make a comparison – as balanced as possible – between science and practice. As way of an introduction to this, I wish to outline some characteristics of scientific research as it has developed since the seventeenth century.

- Scientific research draws borders around the object researched; the phenomenon to be investigated is isolated as much as possible from its surroundings (the more influences there are, the more likely it is that one can be deceived by one's senses).
- Scientific research aims at universal insight. Only statements that are always and everywhere applicable (and which enable one to make predictions) are worthwhile. The development of theories via logic and experiment is required.
- Because scientific research is highly specific in its research aims, it takes note in a thorough and controlled manner of occurring phenomena, forming an antidote to prejudice and hasty conclusions.
- The focus on the phenomenon in itself, however, does lead researchers to not see the network of relations to which the phenomenon belongs. A fragmented view of reality results.
- Generally, valid knowledge makes predictions possible. The extent to which predictions can be made determines the extent to which one is prepared for future occurrence – which is more than a slight advantage.
- One is blind for development. Until recently science regarded change as an illusion. This meant that one of the most important dimensions of human daily life was left out of consideration; namely that we develop from the past via the present towards the future, and that this movement is unrepeatable.

This short survey of the ideas hidden behind science, indicates how easily tensions can occur in its relationship to daily life (and thus with experience). These tensions will become even more clear, if we try to appreciate from which points of view practitioners see, and approach, reality.

Practitioners, in no matter what field, approach problems and tasks facing them, in a way quite different from that of scientific researchers. Not only do the views of reality differ, but also the opinions are obtained by following different routes. Swimming and cycling form perhaps an unexpected but a clear example of what I mean. Swimmers and cyclists do not know (exactly) what they are doing and therefore cannot put their actions into words. They act without (articulated) knowledge of what happens: *...practical wisdom is more truly embodied in action than expressed in rules of action* (Ryle, 1949). This applies to everything made-by-hand, including the social (welfare) services. The actions of practitioners are guided more by (intuitively arising) intentions than by clear, known rules. Rules do exist but they serve to orientate oneself and not as instructions. For example:

A group leader played Risk with three difficult children. The game was recorded on video. Not until she saw the images, did the group leader notice that she was occupied all the time with one specific boy, explaining to him in detail and explicitly the rules of the game. Only then could she support her actions with arguments: the child needed a structure. It is worth mentioning that the boy was very restless and aggressive but nevertheless took part in the whole game continuing to play even when it had become evident that he was going to lose.

Explicit rules and prescribed procedures cannot replace practical insight. Sometimes this aspect to practice leads people to conclude that practical work takes place on a lower level than scientific activity. Such a statement is based, however, on an incorrect impression of what practical activity actually is. Actions are always aimed at objectives. The practitioner's attention is completely absorbed by the particular objectives of his/her actions. The central position of intentionality in practitioner consciousness is called *focal awareness* (Polany, 1967). But since every action takes place under certain circumstances and in certain surroundings, information about these circumstances and surroundings should be present in consciousness, otherwise action cannot take place correctly and smoothly. But attention must not be focused on the context, because in that case one becomes distracted and the action fails. Contextual information does, however, form a background of which one is vaguely aware and in which action is fitted inadvertently; this is called *subsidiary awareness* (op cit). If one does attempt to bring subsidiary awareness into articulated knowledge (concepts and rules), action will become less agile. One can cycle, swim, saw a piece of wood, etc. as long as one does not pay too much attention to how, where or when this is being done.

Practical knowledge not only differs from scientific knowledge, but it is also acquired in a different way. As practical knowledge is not (and should not be) articulated, it cannot be transferred by means of detailed rules. Neither will people learn to swim by being told how to do so, nor can teachers (group leaders) be told how to deal with a certain child. This also applies to the practical uses of scientific research. They too can only be learned by modeling oneself after a gifted practitioner (except perhaps in the case of gifted pupils, but these are few and far between). For example:

A group leader tells that she often prefers to touch children or give them a sign of understanding by means of a gesture. That is often more useful than to approach them with words. In this way the remark or comment remains restricted to the child concerned without the interference of others. It is not possible to do this with all children; some don't like it, with others it doesn't work; it also depends on the circumstances.

Such nuances of practice can only be learned in two ways:
- by experience: i.e. learning by trial and error, or
- by means of examples learned from someone acknowledged to be an appropriate model (anticipatory socialization).

The first way remains restricted to the individual; the knowledge acquired dies out together with the individual. Only if the experience gained is passed on from one (senior teacher) to the other (junior teacher) does the knowledge become:
- shared; not only can the learner make use of the knowledge, but often many different learners gain from one teacher whereby a school is created, turning the activity and insight into common practice or knowledge.
- cumulative; the successors add something to the knowledge of their predecessors whereby insight gains in quality and quantity.

Learning by example means that one has to submit to an authority; in the first instance perhaps even in a rather submissive manner. Not the learning of (abstract) rules matters, but practitioners need to learn the tricks, i.e. to absorb the insights present with the teacher, but which cannot (or only can be partly) expressed (Schon, 1983).

All this leads the scientific researcher to the conclusion that the practitioner's view of the world differs from his/her own. The practitioner sees, to use a metaphor, no trees but this tree under these specific circumstances. As far as s/he knows something in general about trees, s/he mixes this knowledge with experience. The experiences may be gained here and now, or in the past. Clearly practical vision leads to a characteristic combination of advantages and disadvantages:
- Practical activity is organized in fields. Practitioners concentrate on a subject, but do not clearly circumscribe their activity. Their thought is flooded with subsidiary associations and therefore provides a broad perspective. Justice is done to the structure of the particular situation.
- However, the practitioner is not clearly aware of his/her associations. Valuable knowledge does develop, but it remains difficult to articulate and transfer. The

danger arises that one becomes flooded by a bulk of information (leading to hasty, unjustifiable conclusions).

- Practitioners are directed very much towards the actual here and now; they have little interest in truth in general.
- The fields of practice develop. The time dimension determines for a large part the practitioners' view of reality. The world is seen as changeable and makeable. Improvising and experimenting is more important than are scientifically justifiable procedures grounded in specific knowledge.

Having looked at science and practice apart, I now wish to direct my attention to the *relationship between science and practice*. This relation is mostly referred to as *technology*. The term alludes to the relationship between technical knowledge and technical practice. In the course of time, however, technology has been construed more and more to offer a model that prescribes how the relation ought to be between all forms of scientific knowledge and action. We shall see, however, that this opinion is not tenable and in fact is incorrect on at least two points.

Technology and professionalism

Because scientific statements strive to be universally valid, they are somewhat out of their element when one is addressing a single concrete situation. Scientific statements are to some extent applicable to the unique situation, but not completely so; according to an often heard remark: They have to be translated. The translation proceeds via technology. Technology is derived from theory, made available to practitioners in the form of "science based technology" (Ziman, 1984). One-way traffic is involved here; science guides technology, which in turn determines the actions of practitioners. Theory supposedly also provides insight into the cause of possible problems and insight into the way they can be solved. The model of thought: if one knows how a machine works, one also knows why it does not work and what to do about it.

The model which gives hierarchical priority to science appears, when further examined, to be too simplistic. The history of the relationship between technology, industrialization, and science reveals more a joint venture between the three factors than a hierarchical relationship: "At the present time advocacy of the hierarchical model is in a steep decline, and among those in the serious study of science and technology it may already be defunct" (Barnes & Edge, 1982). The concept of technology wherein science determines practice is the first of two misconceptions which I promised at the end of the previous paragraph to explore. I propose to keep this concept of a joint venture firmly in mind.

The idea that the only way theory and practice can go hand in hand is via Technology, is the second misconception I wish to discuss. In all cultures institutions exist with the task of storing, guarding, and processing acquired knowledge; this was the case already long before modern science began its stormy development. Knowledge irrevocably leads to action; via the acquisition of knowledge an image of the world is created, on the basis of which plans of action are made. Technology is only one possible way of getting from (theoretical-technical) knowledge to (rules with regard to) practical action. Another way to collect and store knowledge is to be classified under the concept *professional*. In professional knowledge the relationship between knowledge and practice is conceived to be unreliable, or at best prescientific, thus differing fundamentally from the theoretical-technical model.

Since ancient times physicians and (more particularly) lawyers have been considered to be professionals. Lawyers avail themselves in their work of (theoretical) knowledge, i.e. of jurisprudence. That knowledge is applied again and again (jurisdiction) and is re-adjusted on the basis of new experiences and/or changed circumstances (legislation). Lawyers help people on the basis of knowledge collected by the professional group. In order to carry out and complete their tasks, lawyers considered it to be their right to define their professional role more or less as they see fit. They have acquired a *social mandate* (Hughes, 1971); their profession has became *a major profession* (Glazer, 1974) and a source of power and influence (Freidson, 1986).

Only in our century have paramedicals, psychologists, and social workers (to mention only a few) been added to the category professionals. These practitioners have gained professional status because the demands made on workers within these fields are about the same as those met by lawyers. Unlike most professions, no uniform products are turned out or are services offered which can easily be regulated in standard procedures. One is expected to have the necessary knowledge and experience at one's disposal to be able to offer assistance under varying circumstances and via complex combinations of action. The necessary knowledge and skills are acquired by means of a lengthy (specialized) training. Professional activities in these sectors cannot be planned in detail; a great deal of improvisation is needed to skillfully deal with the ever changing demands made of these professions. Practitioners need a wide margin of decision-making competence. Clearly defined, rigid objectives are out of the question; the same can be said of standard actions prescribed by *higher ups* in the professional organization. The professional is expected, in the carrying out of his/her profession, to link knowledge and experience in a vision of his/her own which does justice to the actual situation where in help is needed. Professional knowledge consists clearly of more elements than scientific knowledge alone; elements which matter include:

- situational knowledge (i.e. knowledge grounded in the concrete situation wherein help is being asked);

- an ability to make a diagnosis (i.e. to be able to develop an informed vision of the specific situation);
- action which provides help at the right time (i.e. which cannot be repeated under exactly the same circumstances).

I can now point clearly to the differences between professional and technological activity. Technology is derived from theoretical, i.e. codified (or "certain") knowledge. Thus it prescribes frames of reference and action steps: If one wants to repair a machine one can better adhere to the instructions. Professional activity is based on knowledge, but this knowledge is of a different kind. To clearly describe this distinction two concepts are very helpful: focal awareness and subsidiary awareness. In science (and to a certain extent also in technology) emphasis is put on data from which all subsidiary associations have, as much as possible, been removed. For example in a correlation between two bare phenomena A en B (bare because the specific circumstances have, as much as possible, been excluded), the phenomena are focussed upon as contextless. In professional activity, on the other hand, subsidiary associations are important. Professional knowledge originates from within a broad range of possible points of attention. Action is based on a mixture of verified theories and practical experiences (or ideas from hearsay). In short, the knowledge is personal and effective because it is integrated into the professional's life. The professional's view of a situation and his/her plans are not based on scientifically guaranteed information but on combinations of life experiences with all sorts of indirect observations playing a role.

Social and welfare education

Some roots to the tension between science and practice have now been exposed. This tension can even be felt in the field of engineering, despite the fact that mechanics have been at the core of the scientific tradition since the sixteenth century. In technical matters, however, many of the original tensions have been absorbed in a joint venture where theory and practice alternatively take the lead. Why can we speak of a joint venture in the relationship between social science and social welfare? Precisely the absence of such a relation is the cause of the large-scale discontent among teachers and welfare workers. Only seldomly can one recognize one's own experience in the results of scientific research. Most theory is experienced as being of little relevance. Why is the gap between social science and education so much bigger than that between natural science and engineering? Two arguments can be put forward.

Classical science keeps its distance from concrete reality; it sees a collection of trees instead of a wood or a tree. Science looses sight in this way of everyday reality; its knowledge is externally structured. Repercussions of distant external structuring are to be found in the professional advice for treatment. Clients are examined and put into categories (neurotic, depressive, etc.). Most secondary associations are lost. But subsidiary associations are necessary preconditions for determining the appropriate action steps. The practitioner needs to take considerably more influences into account (which often have to be spotted out of the corner of the eye) than just those narrowly defined as belonging to the phenomenon under attention. S/he can do next to nothing with the categorical knowledge of (scientific) tunnel vision. S/he requires knowledge which is genuinely applicable to a concrete situation. This is true of all practical work, but especially of social welfare and education where the practitioner has to deal with: (i) whole networks of (often hidden) associations; and (ii) subsidiary thoughts and associations in their client's minds. Furthermore, in education and welfare clients are often highly reactive, i.e. they react to even the slightest stimulus emanating from the professional interaction. Professional action thus becomes implied in client conduct; that conduct thus becomes virtually incalculable, i.e. difficult to put into laws and impossible to predict. Much more than with physics and technology, the processes involved take place rapidly and can change from one moment to the next. Teachers and welfare workers know this very well. Circumstances change quickly; likewise *how* something is experienced, the attitudes, and conduct of those concerned, changes. If regularities are found, they often have a short *half-value time* (Cronbach, 1975). Therefore, any theory designed on the basis of observed regula- rities, quickly loses its significance. If one sticks to such a theory, misunderstandings and conflicts arise. The theory ends up imposing an outlook which does not match reality (Lynch, 1985).

The above mentioned conclusions have considerable significance for the education and training of practitioners. Traditional training supposes that valid theories or models can be transferred without much concern for practic. The reliability of the theory and its relevancy to practice is taken for granted. The content of training emphasizes ideologies and theories about the world instead of stressing experiences within it. We have seen that even in the technological sector this principle leads to tension. When it concerns human relations, even less reliability and relevance ensues. There is, in that case, substantially more tension between theory and practice.

The danger exists that this tension may become a structural element to education and training. This will be the case if education and training, as often happens, go their own separate ways. The result will be that:

- the theories offered will inadequately reflect what is going on; they look, so to speak, back to the past and do not form an introduction to what will demanded from practitioners;
- practical experiences will not be regarded as a worthy source of knowledge, and will not be included in the curriculum.

A combination of two undesirable phenomena threatens:
- trainees are confronted with invalid (or only partly valid) theories;
- trainees do not learn under supervision from work experience.

Incumbent to this analysis there is a suggested solution, namely to combine theoretical knowledge (as valid as possible) with practical study. We shall discuss this suggestion in the next section.

Conclusion

There seems to be a wide gap between the knowledge offered during training and the knowledge which one needs to have at one's disposal in practice. Research (Grubben, Stuyts & Van den Dungen, 1990) confirms this impression; education and practice seem to be going their own ways. Trainees are painfully confronted with the fact that the effectiveness of their education is, hereby, greatly reduced. Both in initial training and continuing education the discrepancy between what is learned at school and the demands made by practice looms very large. Herein the teacher's position resembles that of a welfare worker. Both are faced with tasks that can hardly ever be successfully fulfilled with the simple application of theory. Not only formal knowledge, but also creativity, improvisation, and experiential knowledge are needed. For these professional groups, education should not be limited to the mere transfer of formal knowledge. The development of effective and efficient practical expertise is at least as important. This should not, as has often been the case, be allowed to escape the attention of the educational institutions.

Education needs redefining so that formal knowledge and daily experience are attuned to each other and information is recycled from one level to the other:
- education needs to be characterized by interaction between university and practice;
- education should within one institution provide initial training as well as continuing education;
- initial training, in–service work, pedagogical research and continuing education should all be part of an integrated process.

Only an integrated cooperation between learning on the job and the educational institutions can turn around the existing tension which often produces such a negative effect. Well-balanced variation is especially important; in concrete terms such an educational system might encompass:
- an introductory year (in cooperation with the secondary educational institution),
- three years of practice with intensive work guidance and evaluation provided on the job, and
- three years of study.

This to be followed by (a minimum of) three years of work experience after which one chooses between:
- a career in practical work, or
- university (or higher vocational) training for management and advisory functions, or
- university training for a research career.

Such collaboration would require institutional support:
- *working groups* comprising the educational institutions and the organizations providing on-the-job learning would contribute towards effective (further) integration. Instructors would at regular (not too limited) times participate in practitioner work whilst practitioners would participate in the lecturing (as visiting instructors);
- *regional service centres* would be needed to provide information to the school as well as the organizations. This way the educational institutions can develop into *centres of expertise* in possession of practical experience as well as up-to-date theoretical knowledge. These centres of expertise could collect empirical knowledge, purify and integrate it with formal knowledge, and disseminate it;
- the value of scientific data, hypotheses, and theories are traditionally determined by the consensus reached among scientists; in the context described here this *forum* needs to be extended to practitioners. To put it differently, the collection of knowledge of actions and phenomena that take place in (social) practice, can support no hierarchy in which judgements are exclusively made on scientific grounds.

The objectives just outlined form the background of a practically-oriented research project which I am currently involved in. Practically oriented (or service rendering) research tries to remove (or at least decrease) the tension between research and practice (Doets, 1982; Plooij & Van den Dungen, 1985). The aim is to develop social science in such a way that practitioners can understand what is going on and in consequence will be more inclined to make use of the results. To that end the research:
- tries to answer questions which have surfaced in practice;
- develops its methods in the field in close cooperation with practitioners;
- formulates conclusions so that practitioners can work with them.

For the rest, practically oriented research submits to the fundamental demands that all research has to meet (Miles & Huberman, 1984). Thus a cyclic process of observation, reflection and empirical verification lies at its base.

My research question was presented to me by a higher vocational training institute for youth care. Research was required that: (i) would clarify to what extent the institute knew how to realize its objectives; and (ii) would provide solutions to the problems the institute had in realizing those objectives. Within the research project, meanings and interpretations have carried more weight than the analysis of the instrumental relationship between means and objectives (Harré, 1982, Bhaskar, 1982; Lincoln & Guba, 1985). Data has been mainly gathered by means of (direct) observations and open interviews (Grubben et al, 1990). Because of the primary concern for interpretation, the collected information has had to be continually discussed by those for whom it is important (in this case teachers, students, practitioners, and researchers). Only in that way will the data recognizably reflect participants' ideas and desires. Especially since practically–oriented research entails frequent mutual contact there is no reason not to:

- look together systematically for solutions to apparent problems;
- stimulate practice to develop (organisationally) in the desired direction.

The research has been going on for two years and the first results are visible (Stuyts & Grubben, 1990). The most essential conclusions are:

- the transfer of information between university educators and professional practice does indeed leave a lot to be desired,
- there is insufficient methodology available, both for training as well as for the practical work at hand,
- because the qualifications to be met by practitioners are not made clear enough in the training curriculum, the final terms to met are applied arbitrarily.

In the in-service training of students (internships), the tension between education and profession is most evident. The traineeship forms the link between training and profession. Even here (where the interests of education and practice meet) the connection is weak. This is apparent from student accounts as well as from those of supervisors (whether university or in-service based). The mutual exchange of information is incidental and is often (more or less) confidential.

To find solutions for the lack of communication, an innovation process was designed in consultation with those concerned. The data from interviews with teachers, students, workers, and policymakers served as the basis. Within this training scheme a *platform* connecting three domains (education, welfare work, and traineeship) was set up. Regular consultative meetings (the platform) are held during which the course and the direction taken by the research are discussed and when necessary adjusted.

Two years is of course a fairly short period. If the results are compared with the proposed objectives, it is clear that many wishes are still unfulfilled. In the future, for instance, practitioner research will have to be woven into the organizational infrastructure. The best way to do this, is by gradually extending the cooperation between the working groups such that regional service centres will develop. Collaboration with scientific institutions will then inevitably ensue. The many stakeholders who have to be involved in practitioner research form a complicating factor. But this is more than compensated by the fact that practically-oriented research fulfils two crucial needs:

- it arouses interest in the in-service activities under research. The interviews, feedback sessions, discussions of research reports all focus attention on practice;
- it has an exemplary function when scientific research proves directly service-able.

Practice-oriented research dove-tails into innovation; this has the following advantages:
- connections between practice, education, and research are intensified,
- trainees (students) who are unsuitable or insufficiently motivated for practical work can be spotted quickly,
- at the completion of graduate studies the student has had work experience and is more mature,
- the university as research centre has a clearer role and function than is now the case,
- research is integrated in the total social welfare system by means of cooper-ation between various (welfare & educational) institutions,
- the integration of practical research with training provides for the continuous collection of practical knowledge which helps to narrow the gap between theory and practice.
- continuous data collection insures that the insights produced remain up-to-date.

The fragmentation between university and school, as well as between pedagogic research and teaching, is reduced. Furthermore the welfare system is made more dynamic. Only when university level education/research and in-service practice interact, will students be prepared to accept that pedagogics is a three dimensional activity. On the one hand theory can remain up-to-date and on the other hand a *fund of experience* can be built up, systematized and critically evaluated.

The more practical research takes place, the greater the chance that up-coming generations of professionals will learn the skills needed to reflect on their own work and to collect data in consultation with colleagues. An organization (or if desired, a movement) is needed to further the transference of experience and skills. Teacher Research invites people, in educational practice, to reflect on and to develop their talents. Hereby practice gains the attention it deserves; teachers do not merely carry out plans made elsewhere, but act as independent sources of knowledge. Teacher Research sets an example that deserves to be followed throughout the social sector.

Chapter 8

THE DEVELOPMENT OF PROFESSIONAL COMPETENCE AND INTERACTION: NEW GOALS FOR IN-SERVICE TRAINING AND STAFF DEVELOPMENT

Kees van der Wolf and Pascalle Ramaekers,
University of Amsterdam

It is teachers who, in the end, will change the world of the schools by understanding it. (Lawrence Stenhouse, quoted in Rudduck & Hopkins, 1985)

Introduction

During the last several years there has been extensive discussion of the in-service training of teachers in the Dutch primary schools. In general the opinions expressed have been very critical. There seems to be much which stands in need of improvement. We begin this chapter by first taking a brief look at the policy which has been taking shape with regard to in-service training.[1] After a phase in which it took a non-committal position, the Dutch government is trying to come to grips with changes in the primary school. Recently new ground has been broken. In a climate of privatization, deregulation and market ideas, school-administration and schools themselves are being encouraged to decide how in-service training will take place.

Emphasis has been on the strategic and financial aspects of policy. It is obviously advisable to think further about the content of the future in-service training. An attempt in this direction will be made in this chapter. To acquire insight into the professionalization of teachers in the primary school, the profession of the teacher has to be discussed. Being a teacher is a fairly low status job. Teachers do not seem to believe very strongly in their own competence. Social interaction with colleagues seems to contribute little to teacher professional development; teachers do not work much together. On the basis of American and Dutch assessment studies, a number of proposals to stimulate improved in-service training will be formulated. We aim to examine the qualities which in-service training institutions need to possess to be effective. In-service training should, in our opinion, lead to an inquiring attitude which encourages the development of a professional attitude promoting interaction with colleagues and support staff. We will emphasize that in-service training should play an important role in school-based curriculum development. We conclude with a preliminary sketch of an in-service training programme which could be developed in the framework of the "Amsterdams Pedologisch Centrum".

In-service training and in-service training policy in the Netherlands

In the Netherlands, the in-service training of teachers in primary education has only received proper attention in recent years. For a long time, the attitude of the central government was noncommittal. Occasional subsidies were given. This fairly benevolent neglect led to a great variety of in-service training. In 1980 the Dutch Minister of Education decided to formulate annual *in-service training plans*. Anticipating the introduction of the new primary school (in 1985 the previously separate kindergartens for 4-6 year-olds and primary schools for the 6-12 year-olds were integrated), the plan was launched of using in-service training to renew educational practice. In the period 1976-1979 the focus was on school curriculum development. After that, cooperation between kindergarten teachers and primary school teachers was the hot item. Later still, the emphasis was shifted to reading. Teacher Training Colleges for Primary Education developed courses which fit the national innovation policy. Courses were initiated in the fields of emancipation, choosing policy priorities, and information technology. Of all the courses announced half were never given because of a lack of interest. What was on offer was evidently not found to be very attractive.[2] In 1985, with the introduction of the *Salaries Review System in Education (HOS)*, in-service training became a criterion for promotion. If a teacher wanted to become a senior teacher, then s/he had to participate in in-house training. After 1987 the responsibility for the programming of in-service courses shifted from government responsibility to the schools and the teacher training institutes. This meant that people in the field (schools and instructors) had to define their own quality criteria. The government directive *In-service Training in Primary and Secondary Education* (1988) went further in this same line. Autonomy and responsibility for in-service training was devolved to the schools. It was assumed that this would lead schools to become critical customers in the training market place. Government has reduced its role to offering a general policy framework coupled to providing some supervision. School governors and school managements have been obliged to take responsibility for staff in-service training. These school governors and school managements, to fulfill the task required of them, will have to acquire more competence in the training field. The government directive included a plan for, in the future, no longer supplying funds for in-service training to training bodies, but instead to make the funds directly available to the schools. Schools will have a separate budget allocation for in-service training and to develop *Human Resource Management* policies.

"As a minimum norm for the allocation of the budget for in-service training, the budget must be of such a type that in one year, one in five teachers must be able to participate in about forty hours of in-service training. The school becomes the buyer. Through market orientation, profiling and mutual competition, we are attempting to stimulate the quality of in-service training. The transfer of funds from the in-service training institutions to the schools will have to be completed by 1995. For the schools in primary education there is then a sum of 54 million guilders available." (Van Tulder e.a., 1989, p. 5)

A review of the plans for the future of in-service training in the Netherlands reveals that hardly any attention has been paid to the content of the in-service training. The emphasis has been on organizational and legal questions, on problems of coordination and demarcation. Summing up, it can be said that the existing structures are perceived to be unsatisfactory. Courses given by Teacher Training Colleges (PABO's), other teacher training (or comparable institutions), do not make a significant (enough) contribution to the improvement of the quality of education. In line with the ideology of *less government is better government* the Ministry of Education argues that schools and School Boards have been unable to get a sufficient grip on the budgets for in-service training. The government argues in favour of a direct allocation of these funds to the schools. Deregulation is looked upon to be the solution to previous problems. Schools and their governors will supposedly know themselves what is best for themselves. This policy is meant to usher in a new era in in-service training (In-set). Teacher training institutes, school advisory services, national pedagogic centres, institutions for high technical training, universities and private institutions are all supposedly going to compete on the privatized In-set market. The dust clouds are already visible. There will be new opportunities, but also new dangers. There is a chance that in the haste to preserve market share that some stakeholders will turn to the very tried and true programmes which led in the past to dissatisfaction; i.e. old wine (or vinegar?) in new privatized bottles. But the new policy does offer an opportunity to rethink one's attitude to In-set. Before we examine what we consider to be a desirable approach to in-service training, a short sociological discussion of the *profession* teacher will help us to clarify the needs of the target group. Before beginning on In-set curriculum development, one needs to have a clear impression of the learners' situation.

The teaching profession: status, competence, collegial interaction

The examination of salary levels is a good way of assessing the value which society places on a profession. Beginning primary school teachers earn, after taxes and deductions, little more than unemployment benefits. In this, the Netherlands is out of step with the rest of the world. Furthermore, career advancement for teachers takes place very slowly. The maximum salary is only reached around the age of fifty; older teachers are comparatively well paid. It seems, thus, that in the Netherlands the teaching profession is not very highly valued. The professional standing of teaching has, in fact, been eroded. The profession is not seen to be very attractive. Hargreaves (1980), speaking about secondary school teachers, distinguishes three central themes to teachers professional culture: status, competence and relations with colleagues. We believe that much of what he says can be applied to teachers in primary education:

– as we have indicated the level of professional status is fairly low. Teaching is perceived to be a typically female profession (Lortie, 1969, 1975). Because men feel unsure of themselves in a profession which is seen as to be feminine (Adorno, 1965), they will not choose it enthusiastically. Often when men do become teachers they have made a negative choice (nothing else was available). Many women feel a similar ambivalence. In American research, female students at a Teacher Training College were asked if they would want to marry a man who would make the teaching of children up to the age of twelve, his life's work. In general, the response was No. Since women, reputedly, do not make their professional choices so much from a career perspective, they are willing to become teachers.[3] Women are reported to be attracted to the fairly short, practice-orientated initial training. Supposedly the possibility of re-entering teaching once the children have left home also plays a role.

Status is also judged on the basis of the perceived difficulty of a profession. People assume that what one can teach children under twelve is not very difficult. In secondary education the teachers who have studied the most difficult subjects (mathematics, chemistry) enjoy the highest prestige. The difficulty of the subject matter is confused with the difficulty of teaching it;

– the sense of competence of primary school teachers is also problematic. A teacher told Lortie (1975, p. 143): "One just plods along, hoping for the best." Teaching seems to fall far short of what is understood by a profession. Teacher training is noticeably less based on systematic knowledge than is training in the acknowledged professions. We note that in the relationship between the professional and client, engineers lawyers and doctors come into action when the client demands professional help. The client wants something (a house built, a court case won) or has something (a throat infection) and the professional can do something about it. The engineer, lawyer and doctor possess

Van der Wolf & Ramaekers ❖❖❖

professional knowledge in the form of practical expertise, knowledge of jurisprudence, medical techniques. But the relationship between the teacher and pupil is notable for the lack of standard procedures and for the fact that the pupil has not chosen to be helped. It is difficult to determine the knowledge base upon which the practical procedures of the teacher are based. The repertory of behaviours is highly complicated but much less specific. Furthermore pupils are not pedagogically solely in the hands of teachers. Parents, school managements, inspectors, the Ministry, all have their role to play. Teachers are limited to the extent to which they can decide what they should do. They are involved in a network of hierarchic relationships. The Dutch government's mania for organization reinforces this phenomenon. Other professions have much more room to manoeuvre, and greater autonomy.[4] They can establish their own rules. Doctors have their own procedures for admitting novices; they have their trade secrets and their own jurisprudence. Teachers work in an atmosphere of duty, obedience to regulations and dependence on managerial policy. All this has a negative influence on their sense of competence;

– the third theme discussed by Hargreaves concerns the relational network of the teacher. It is a profession where the practitioner often works in isolation. Teachers mostly work alone in the class. Between teachers there is a lack of a pedagogic discourse of consultation. Very little time is set aside for genuine discussion. This inhibits the development of teaching as a profession and makes it very difficult to develop the conceptual system which goes with professionalization. Furthermore, teaching is a profession in which one has to teach oneself. Beginning teachers often receive no help from experienced colleagues which often leads to an intuitive approach. The resulting trial and error method obstructs the growth of a theoretical framework. In result *good teaching* gets ascribed to certain charismatic qualities: You either have it or you haven't. It's not a profession you can learn.

We have focused on the profession of the teacher. Professionalization through in-service training is, given the nature of the profession, far from a self-evident option. The appreciation by society and by teachers of teaching is obviously relatively low. There is no esoteric knowledge and formalized skill. We will examine these considerations once again later in this chapter when we examine the consequences our findings have for the development of in-service training. In the next section we will examine relevant developments in Dutch primary education.

Problems and developments in Dutch primary education

The issues in Dutch education do not differ much from those elsewhere. When the Minister of Education became worried about the nature and scale of criticism of his educational policy, he asked the Organization for Economic Cooperation and Development (OECD) to assess Dutch education. In the resulting *Review of Educational Policy in the Netherlands*, three examiners (from West Germany, Sweden and the USA) gave what they saw to be a comprehensive picture of the Dutch situation. Many people in the Netherlands were surprised by the conclusions. Dutch education was judged to be relatively good, to very good. The level attained by Dutch pupils is, in comparison to elsewhere, not at all that bad. Furthermore, by expending six and a half percent of the gross national product on education, Holland was comparatively speaking quite generous. The deregulation policy of the government met with the full approval of the OECD. They supported more autonomy for the schools. It was noted that much bureaucratic resistance would have to be overcome. Nevertheless, there were a number of difficulties. The integration of kindergartens into the primary schools has not gone very well. Teachers displayed a clear lack of professional self-awareness and professional interaction. Many part-time teachers did not have the opportunity to work with others. Dutch teachers evidently teach almost always on their own. Insufficient time is devoted to developing school policy, to discussing alternative ways of working or to generating frequent and accurate feedback. There is too little in-service training. The starting salaries are too low. The primary schools are stretched to the limits; regulations have become petrified. School management leaves much to be desired. There is an atmosphere of dissatisfaction.

At more or less the same time that the OECD study came out, a number of Dutch experts commissioned by a Dutch teachers' union (ABOP) put forward their proposals to make teaching more attractive. Their suggestions:

– teachers should not stand alone in front of their class; they should be responsible together for clusters of pupils. Cooperation between teachers needs to be promoted.
– performance appraisal should be used to promote the quality of in class teaching.
– schools should be free to develop their own financial policies.
– education needs more middle level managers with appropriate salaries.
– teaching positions need to be differentiated: the distinction between junior and senior teachers needs to be implemented.
– school management needs to become more professional.
– more task differentiation and more career opportunities are needed. Education must find ways to hold onto talented practitioners.
– labor restrictions which hinder teaching must be revised.

Both the OECD report and the ABOP study point to the importance of in-service training and professionalization. The time seems to be ripe for professionalizing teaching and for developing new working practices. In the next section we will examine some key current issues in in-service training.

In-service training in the Netherlands: a problem area

In our introduction we suggested that there were reasons to be concerned about in-service training in the Netherlands. Many teachers are supposedly unhappy about what they have experienced. Remarkably enough, however, this complaint did not emerge in an extensive evaluation study of Dutch in-service training completed by Van Tulder, Veenman and Roelofs in 1989. The teachers seemed to be very satisfied with the in-service training they had experienced. In conclusion, the authors state: in-service training makes a difference. However if we take a more detailed look at the data, quite another picture emerges. According to the trainees, less then half of the in-service instructors take the practical problems of the teacher in the classroom into account. The possibilities to implement what has been learned in the courses is considered to be quite low. Application in practice is, in general, not considered to be easily possible. In addition, there is insufficient course follow-up and feedback. What then are trainees actually happy about? Surely these are devastating criticisms? Perhaps Festinger's theory of cognitive dissonance can help us to understand the results. People have the tendency to justify retrospectively a choice already made. They do not easily admit that they made the wrong decision. This is perhaps also true of teachers in in-service training. Following a course requires time and effort. If one gives a course a negative evaluation, one admits that one has wasted a substantial amount of time. In general, people do not like to do this. Furthermore, we should bear in mind that the trainees fill in assessment forms in a situation of potential judgment anxiety. Trainees probably find it difficult to be critical of course instructors *who were really doing their best, and who couldn't help it either.* It turns out that the courses really did not go half so well. The following picture emerges: current in-service training is insufficiently based on the teaching process itself and the role of the teacher in it. Although trainees fill-in post-course happiness sheets contentedly enough, the in-service training is not thought to be of much use in the classroom. Regrettably in the in-service training that is on offer, the possibility is overlooked of drawing on the teachers' own capacity for in-school (and/or classroom) innovation. Teachers' lack of awareness of the potential for change, which can be achieved by reflecting themselves on their own practical situation, stops them from being critical and from coming up with ideas leading to improvement. On the contrary, teachers are continually confronted with changes imposed by others (especially, central government). Teachers are little aware of what their own share could be in determining the structure and content of in-service training. The in-service training which has been realized in the Netherlands has provided little improvement in this sorry state of affairs.

What is required from in-service training

In the meta-analysis of the in-service training literature carried out by Showers, Joyce and Bennett (1987) a number of important conclusions emerge. For long almost all publications in the field have been descriptively orientated and have focused on course (training) content. Only a limited number of publications report any empirical research into training (results). In recent years we have seen an increase in research reports which examine how teaching skills can be best taught. Attention is now being paid to the extent to which courses have an effect. Resulting from this research is the finding that In-set must do more than just interest teachers in new teaching methods and skills. *"What the teacher* thinks *about teaching determines what the teacher* does *when teaching"* (p. 78). For the design of in-service training this means that aiming only for a transfer of knowledge will lead to a low magnitude of effect. But if the transfer of knowledge is supplemented by demonstrations and opportunities to practice new skills, as well as ample feedback, the effect rises by a factor of three. Furthermore, when there is expert or colleague back-up, the effect is even stronger. It is clear that back-up support, given during the implementation of what has been learned, is very important to effectiveness. The authors state:*" ...the message is an optimistic one, since it appears that the coaching process enables nearly all teachers to sustain practice and gain executive control over a large range of curricular and instructional practices"* (p. 86).

On the basis of their study Van Tulder et al (1989) come up with a number of design characteristics for good in-service training:

- in-service training needs to be orientated to practice; in-service training has to link up with the practical problems of teachers and the way the teacher functions in the school-as-organization;
- when course content is practical and immediately usable, one maximizes the chance that what was learned will also be applied;
- therefore in in-service training the emphasis should be on skills objectives, with knowledge and attitude objectives related the skills goals;
- this means more input into the structure of the course is needed from the students and more skills practice needs to be attained so that training will be attuned to the desires and needs of the participants;
- finally, course effectiveness is related to the presence of training components identified by Joyce and Showers (1980, 1988). In in-service training courses teachers need to:
  1. study and accept the theory or rationale on which the teaching skills to be learned are based,
  2. learn by observation and demonstration,
  3. be able to practice and apply new ideas/skills in safe situations (for example

through role playing or simulation) and
4. receive structured feedback and back-up (coaching).

For in-service training to be effective trainers need to:

– be concrete and purposefully prepared;
– not only set aside time for the preparation of course content, but also for mastering the didactics of training (for example, to learn to work with adult groups, to react skillfully to differing adult learning styles, etc.);
– have a solid insight into in-school practice in order to be aware of the possibilities and capabilities for innovation present in schools.

Thus, in one's didactic approach to in-service training one needs to take into account that In-set is a form of adult education. In effective in-service training the following components are present: (i) adequate information, (ii) skill demonstration, (iii) opportunity to practice what is learned, and (iv) expert and colleague feedback. Below we discuss a proposal for an in-service training which (we hope) fulfills the formulated criteria.

Principles for designing an in-service training

In-service training of teachers faces many problems both in the Netherlands and abroad. Many of these problems are directly related to the characteristics of the teaching profession which were discussed above. The development of a professional identity has been a slow process. We see both in the report of the Dutch Teachers' Union (ABOP) and in the OECD report that a serious lack of professional self-awareness persists. Even worse, the in-service training which is on offer appears to not link up with in-service problems. (Van Tulder et al., 1989). With an eye to developing a more suitable in-service training, two important factors need to be examined. In the first place, a strategy needs to be developed which will promote the professional development of teachers. The authors believe that systematic research into one's own practice can contribute to the improvement of one's professional attitude. In the reports mentioned above it was pointed out that the teaching profession had developed an insufficient level of professional interaction. Teacher development has too often taken place in isolation. Therefore in-service training has to be aimed at strengthening team work and in the formulation of in-school policy. These two aspects of in-service training are developed further below.

Development of professional competence

In 1975 Stenhouse argued that in a professionalized practical situation there must be a research process. Good education is research; an inquiring attitude leads to good teaching. In his An *Introduction to Curriculum Research and Development* he asserted:

- the teacher's professional self-image and conditions of work will have to change (p. 142);
- the commitment to systematic questioning of one's own teaching as a basis for development (is essential for educational advance) (p. 144);

and

- the outstanding characteristic of the extended professional is a capacity for autonomous professional self development through systematic self-study, through the study of the work of other teachers and through the testing of ideas by classroom research procedures (p. 144).

Nias and Groundwater-Smith (1989) have elaborated on the fundamental principles of in-service training based on teacher inquiry. Students must, they argue, be spurred on to take a critical, constructive stance with regard to their professional practice.[5] Teachers must be helped, in the context of in-service training, to select adequate measures which link up with the conclusions of their own studies. Furthermore during the implementation of changes based upon teacher inquiry, (facilitator) back-up needs to be supplied.

We start thus from the following assumptions:

- under suitable conditions teachers have the capacities to undertake valid and reliable inquiry into the various aspects of their practical situation;
- however, they do not usually have the analytical and methodological skills to carry out effective research. Teachers need to have the possibility to develop these skills;
- the subjects chosen for research can be derived from course content. However it is also possible that teachers themselves introduce research themes (see Nias's article);
- on the basis of one's own and other trainees' research teachers can generalize their results to obtain theories of practice which clarify their situation. These theories can then lead to action steps;
- however, teacher inquiry does not always have to lead to action. Professional Inquiry is not a synonym for Action Research, although these two are often related to each other (see Nias);
- when teachers are in control of their own teaching and can develop their own knowledge of practice, the differences between teachers and experts (the infamous silencers) will be minimal.
- the development of criteria for measuring the effects of inquiry in in-service courses requires attention. There is a lack of accepted criteria for assessing teacher inquiry;
- teachers need back-up, to help them reach consensus on the (practical) conclusions of their research, and to implement inquiry into their professional practice.

For the facilitation of in-service inquiry the basic principles just stated mean that one must:

- be able to select and teach research methods which are easy to use in the field. One must also be capable of laying down criteria and adapting them to the assessment of school orientated tasks, even if use is being made of methods of data collection which are not characteristic for experimental, pre-test/post-test tradition and, thus, are not scientifically recognized (!);
- be prepared to collect information and carry out research which is related to the interests of teachers;
- be able and ready to find one's way about in the teaching system as a whole. One will have to maintain contacts with both the management of the local educational institutions and representatives of the local educational policy. One will also have to maintain contacts in the educational sector;
- be able to avoid cursory methods of working. One has to see the teachers as colleagues who are able to reflect on their own practical situation. That reflection will lead to a usable and generalizable theory of practice.

The development of professional interaction

Carr & Kemmis (1986) regard *the teacher as researcher movement* as individualistic. In their opinion, the working methods are insufficiently in accordance with school-based curriculum development. Les Bell (Chapter 4) has gone extensively into the importance of attuning teachers' professional development to the policies of the school. He has also pointed out the dangers; school-based or school-focused thinking assumes that schools can adequately express their needs, and that there are sufficient resources in schools to carry out change. This is often not the case. Bell has rightly pointed out that innovation in schools is a complicated process in which internal and external resources need to be carefully attuned to each other. School faculties, school management as well as institutions for in-service training will have to work together on this. In what Bell calls *the policy-based professional approach to development*, the desires and interests of the school staffs, of sub-groups in those staffs and of individual teachers are taken into account in the choice of in-service training. This links up with the recommendations of the ABOP (see above) in which the plea is made for the creation of middle management functions where the distinction was made between junior and senior teachers and where the introduction of task differentiation and career possibilities for teachers was encouraged. To achieve all this it will be necessary to:

- develop in-service training packages in close cooperation between in-service training institutions and schools (including parents and the competent authorities). However, it must be clear to those involved what financial resources are actually available;

- help schools in the context of in-service training when the need for change has been translated into a diagnosis which reflects in a coherent fashion the problems the participants want to work on. Distinctions will need to be made between individual, sub-group and faculty interests;
- establish regular contacts between in-service instructors and teachers, especially when the school or the teacher is still unsure if it (s/he) should commit itself (her/himself) to the inquiry approach;
- undertake research at the level of the school faculty which contribute to the development of shared technical understandings. Such research can raise teacher professionalism and contribute to analytical capacity. This in turn can form an important contribution to school development and school policy.

The representatives of in-service training institutions need to possess the following expertise:
- be able to support in-service research teams;
- be able to carry out needs analyze in school contexts;
- possess (expert) knowledge or be able to arrange for qualified informants in the fields chosen by the schools.

A preliminary plan for in-service training

A number of basic principles for effective in-service training have been described in this chapter. In this final section a short sketch of a possible strategy is provided. On an annual basis, fifty-four million guiders (± 17 million pounds) will be available in Holland for in-service training in primary education. How can this money best be used?

We would propose to make it known to the schools that we adhere to the principles sketched above. Our in-school training catalogue, distributed to school managements and school faculties, would make our position clear. If schools liked what was on offer, we would investigate on the basis of a needs analysis whether cooperation was desirable. The working method proposed by Bell (in this volume) would be of great use. If agreement was reached, then we would propose that for one year a group of ten teachers would be secunded to work one and a half day per week together on an in-school inquiry project. Preferably, the participants would all come from one single school. The content of their meetings would be grounded in the practical research (based on written observations, log books, document analyses) carried out in the classrooms and school(s). The trainer would provide theoretical and methodological input. The teachers would be encouraged to study some theoretical and methodological subjects themselves. To this end a well-equipped library must be made available wherever the course is held. The participants would, with the use of a collectively chosen theme, observe each other in the classroom. Video-recordings would be made. The analysis of these video recordings would figure in the course meetings. The data collected would be systematically discussed. This data would be recorded in research reports which would then form the basis for assessment. During the course the participants would increasingly coach each other. Role playing and simulations could be employed to encourage feedback.

The development of in-class didactic skills would be the crux to the plan. The role of the teacher in the classroom and in the school would come in for (re-) examination. This form of in-service training would lead to an inquiring stance which encourages professionalism and stimulates the quality of collegial inter-action. This ought to lead to an increased understanding of the teacher's practical situation and to more professional self-awareness whereby professional inter-action would be improved.

Have we succeeded in describing an important task for the years to come for the "Amsterdams Pedologisch Centrum"?

Notes

1. For a description of Dutch policy in this field we refer the reader to Van Wieringen (in this volume).
2. Doornbos (1986) points out that this mania for organization on the part of the Ministry interfered in an undesirable manner with the schools' own advisory procedures. The Ministry interfered in in-service training, because dismissals in the Teacher Training Institutes threatened. By giving in-service training tasks to these institutions less teachers had to be dismisses.
3. Which is not to say that there are no women who have careers in this position.
4. For this theme, we refer you to the article by Van den Dungen (in this volume).
5. Harrison (1962) gives a good description of the relationship between resistance to change and defective conceptual systems among teachers. In thi s still topical article, he sets forth how conceptual frameworks can contribute to adequate teaching.

BIBLIOGRAPHY

Abercrombie, M.L.J. (1960). *The Anatomy of Judgement: An investigation into the processes of perception and reason.* Harmondsworth: Penguin.

Adorno, Th.W. (1965). Tabus über dem Lehrerberuf. In Th. W. Adorno (ed.), *Erziehung zur Mündigkeit.* Frankfurt am Main: Suhrkamp.

Altrichter, H. & Posch, P. (1989). Does the grounded theory approach offer a guiding paradigm for teacher research? *Cambridge Journal of Education,* 19:1, 21-32.

Arfwedson, G. (1985). *School Codes and Teachers' Work. Three Studies on Teachers Work Contexts.* Malmø: Liber.

Argyris, C. (1971). *Management and Organizational development.* London: McGraw-Hill.

Argyris, C. and Schon, D.A. (1976). *Theory in Practice: Increasing professional effectiveness.* San Franciso: Jossey-Bass.

Armstrong, J.Scott. (1982). Strategies for Implementing Change: An Experiential Approach. *Group & Organization Studies,* Vol. 7, no. 4, December.

Audit Commission (1989). *Assuring Quality in Education: The Role of Local Authority Inspectors and Advisers.* Audit Commission for England and Wales.

Barnes, B. & Edge, D. (eds.) (1982). *Science in context: Readings in the sociology of science.* Milton Keynes: The open University Press.

Baudrillard, Jean. (1990). *Cool Memories.* London: Verso.

De Bedrijvige School. Een visie op het onderwijs van de toekomst. (1989). Amsterdam: ABOP.

Bell, G.H. (1985). INSET: five types of collaboration and consultancy. *School Organisation.* Vol. 5, no. 3.

Bell, L.A. (1986). An Investigation of a New Role in Schools: The Case of the TVEI Co-ordinator. In T. Simpkins (ed.), *Research in the Management of Secondary Education.* Sheffield City Polytechnic Papers in Educational Management.

Bell, L.A. (1988a). *Management Skills in Primary Schools.* London: Routledge.

Bell, L.A. (ed.) (1988b). *Appraising Teachers in Schools.* London: Routledge.

Bell, L.A. (1991). *Managing Teams in Secondary Schools.* London: Routledge.

Berg, G. v.d., Harskamp, E.G., Prins, J.B.A. en Wolfgram, H.P. (1986). *Het functioneren van onderwijsbegeleiding op de basisschool*. Groningen: RION.

Bhaskar, R. (1978). Emergence, explanation and emancipation. In P.F. Secord (ed.), *Explaining social behavior: Consciousness, behaviour and social structure*. Hassocks: The Harvester Press.

Billings, D.E. (1977). The Nature and Scope of Staff Development in Institutions of Higher Education. In T. Elton and K. Simmonds (eds.), *Staff Development in Higher Education*. Society for Research into Higher Education.

Bradley, H. (1988). Partnership in the development of school management. In C. Poster and C. Day (eds.), *Partnership in Education Management*. London: Routledge.

Branston (1986). *TRIST - The Branston Proposal*. Draft for Discussion at Academic Board, 14 april 1986.

Branston (1986a). *Branston TRIST (Teachers as Experts)*. Launch Pack, May 1986.

Branston (1986b). *Staff Bulletin. TRIST update*, 23.6.86.

Buchmann, M. (1984). Role over Person. Morality and authenticity in teaching. *Teachers College Record*, 87, 529-543.

Bungard, K. and Bell, L.A. (1988). *Staff Development in Schools*. [mimeograph] Education Department: University of Warwick.

Burgess, Robert. (1982). *Fieldresearch: Its sourcebook and fieldmanual*. London: Allen & Unwin.

Caluwé, L. de, Marx, E.C.H. & Petri, M.W. (1988). *Schooldevelopment, Models & Change*. Leuven: Acco.

Carr, W. & Kemmis, S. (1986). *Becoming Critical: Education, Knowledge and Action Research*. London: Falmer Press.

Carson, T. & Couture, J.C. (eds.) (1988). *Collaborative Action Research: Experience and reflections*. Improvements of Instruction Series, Monograph No 18, Alberta Teachers' Association.

Carter, J. and Bell, L.A. (1987). *Identifying Professional Development Needs: A Report of a Research Project*. Education Department: University of Warwick.

Clark, C. and Peterson, P. (1986). Teachers' Thought Processes. In: M. Witrock (ed.), *Handbook of Research on Teaching, 3rd ed*. New York: McMillan Publishing Comp.

Cohen, L. and Manion, M. (1980). *Research Methods in Education*. Beckenham: Croom Helm.

Connelly, F.M. and Clandinin, D.J. (1985). The Cyclic Temporal Structure of Schooling. Paper presented at Symposium on Classroom Studies of Teachers. Canada: Personal Knowledge, OISE.

Cormier, W.H. and Cormier, L.S. (1979). *Interviewing Strategies for Helpers; a guide to assessment, treatment and evaluation*. Monterey CA: Brooks/Cole.

Cowan, B. and Wright, N. (1990). Two Million Days Lost. *Education*, 2 February, 117-118.

Cronbach, L.J. (1975). Beyond the two disciplines of scientific psychology. *American Psychologist*, 30, 245-257.

Dadds, M., PhD in progress, Cambridge Institute of Education.

Dalin, P. (1989). *Organisatieontwikkeling in school en onderwijs*. Alphen aan de Rijn: Samsom.

Day, C. (1979). *Classroom-based in-service teacher education: The development and evaluation of a client-centered model* [doctoral thesis]. Brighton, Engeland: University of Sussex.

Day, C. (1981). *Classroom-based in-service teacher education: The development and evaluation of a client-centered model.* Occasional Paper No. 9. Brighton: University of Sussex.

Day, C. (1985). Professional Learning and Researcher Intervention. *British Educational Research Journal,* Vol. 11, no. 2.

Day, C. (1990a). In-Service as Consultancy: The Evaluation of a Management Programme for Primary School Curriculum Leaders. In C. Aubrey (ed.), *Consultancy in the United Kingdom* (49-75). Lewes: The Falmer Press,.

Day, C. (1990b). Managing Curriculum Development at Branston School and Community College. In C. March, C. Day, L. Hanney & G. McCutcheon (Eds.), *Re-conceptualising School-Based Curriculum Development (140-171).* Lewes: The Falmer Press.

Day, C., Whitaker, P. and Wren, D. (1987). *Appraisal and Professional Development in Primary Schools.* Milton Keynes: Open University Press.

Department of Education and Science (1972). *Teacher Education and Training* (The James Report). Her Majesties Stationary Office (HMSO).

DES (1977). *Education in Schools: A Consultative Document.* HMSO.

DES (1983). *Circular 3/83: The In-Service Training Grant Scheme.* HMSO.

DES (1985). *Better Schools.* HMSO.

DES (1986). *Circular 6/86: Local Authority Training Grant Scheme.* HMSO.

DES (1987). *The Education (School Teachers' Pay and Conditions of Employment) Order.* HMSO.

DES (1989). *The Implementation of the Local Authority Training Grant Scheme (LEATGS): A Report on the First Year of the Scheme by H M Inspectors.* HMSO.

Doets, C. (1982). *Praktijk en onderzoek; wetenschap in wisselwerking met praktisch handelen.* Amersfoort: De Horstink.

Doornbos, K. (1986). De verzorgingsstructuur van het onderwijs. In J.A. van Kemenade, N.A.J. Lagerweij, J.M.G. Leune, & J.M.M. Ritzen (eds.), *Onderwijs: bestel en beleid 1.* Groningen: Wolters-Noordhoff.

Ebbutt, D. (1982). Educational Action Research: Some general concerns and specific quibbles, *Teacher-Pupil Interaction and the Quality of Learning Project Schools Council Programme 1* (Cambridge Institute of Education).

Eisner, E.W. (1979). *The Educational Imagination.* London: Collier Macmillan.

Eisner, E.W. (1984). Can education research inform educational practice? *Phi Delta Kappan* 65, 7, 447-52.

Elbaz, F. (1983). *Teacher Thinking. A Study of Practical Knowledge.* New York: Nichols.

Elbaz, F. (1990). Knowledge and Discourse: The Evolution of Research on Teacher Thinking. In C. Day, M. Pope and P. Denicolo (eds.), *Insights into Teacher Thinking and Action.* Lewes: The Falmer Press.

Elliott, J. (1976-7). Developing hypotheses about classrooms from teachers' practical constructs: A account of the work of the Ford Teaching Project. *Interchange,* 7:2, 2-21.

Elliot, J. (1977). Conceptualising relationships between researcher/evaluation procedures and in-service teacher education. *British Journal of In-Service Education,* 4, 102-183.

Elliott, J. (1978). *Who Should Monitor School Performance?* [Mimeo]. Cambridge, England: Cambridge Institute of Education.

Elliott, J. (1980). The Theory and Practice of Educational Action Research. *Classroom Action Research Network Bulletin* No 4 (Cambridge Institute of Education).

Elliott, J. (1987) *Onderzoekend Onderwijzen.* Hoevelaken: CPS Publicaties.

Elliott, J. (1987). Educational theory, practical philsophy and action research. *British Journal of Educational Studies,* 35:2, 149-169.

Elliott, J. (1989a). *Studying the school curriculum through insider research: Some dilemmas.* Centre for Applied Research in Education, University of East Anglia, mimeo.

Elliott, J. (1989b). Teacher evaluation and teaching as a moral science. In M.L. Holly & C. McLoughlin (eds.), *Perspectives on Teacher Professional Development.* London: Falmer Press.

Eraut, M. (1972). *In-service education for innovation.* Occasional Paper 4, N.C.E.T.

Eraut, M. (1977). In-Service Courses: their structure and functions. In C. Richards (ed.), *New Contexts for Teaching, Learning and Curriculum Studies.* Leicester, England: Association for the Study of the Curriculum.

Eraut, M. (1982). What is learned in in-service education and how? A knowledge use perspective. *British Journal of In-Service Education..*

Fellows, A. (1989). Identifying and Meeting INSET Needs: Some Thoughts for INSET Co-ordinators. In *Sharing INSET Ideas.* Warwickshire County Council Education Department, pp 41-43.

Fillmore, C. (1976). The need for frame semantics in linguistics. *Statistical Methods in Linguistics.* Stockholm: Skriptor.

Flower, Linda. (1985). *Problem Solving Strategies for Writing,* 2nd edition. New York: Harcourt Brace Jovanovich.

Freidson, E. (1986). *Professional powers: The social structure of medicine.* Chicago: Chicago University Press.

Fullan, M. (1982). *The Meaning of Education Change.* New York: Teachers College Press.

Galesloot, Louis, & Ten Brinke, Steven. (1988). Kunnen een leraar en een buitenstaander samenwerken bij onderwijsvernieuwing in de klas? In H. Letiche (Ed.), *Zelf evaluatie.* Assen: Van Gorcum.

Georgiades, N.J. and Phillimore, L. (1975). The Myth of the Hero Innovator and Alternative Strategies for Organisational Change. In C.C. Keirnan and F.P. Woodford (eds.), *Behaviour Modification with Severely Retarded.* Amsterdam: Elseview Excerpta Medica.

Glazer, N. (1974). Schools of minor professions. *Minerva,* 346, 116-127.

Gray, H.L. (ed.) (1988). *Management Consultancy in Schools.* London: Cassell.

Grubben, L., Stuyts, M. & Dungen, M.G.M. van den. (1990). interviewing: a scientific road to subjective experience. Lecture delivered at The 1990 Principles Congress, Amsterdam.

Grundy, S. (1983). Action Research. In A. Pitman et al (eds.), *Educational Enquiry: Approaches to research.* Victoria, Australia: Deakin University Press.

Grundy, S. and Kemmis, S. (1982). Educational action research in Australia: The state of the art. In S. Kemmis (ed.), *The Action Research Reader.* Victoria, Australia: Deakin University Press.

Hall, J. (1988). *Introduction.* Local Education Authorities Project. Management in Education INSET Initiative. BBC.

Handal, G. and Lauvås, P. (1987). *Promoting Reflective Teaching: Supervision in Action.* Milton Keynes: SRHE/Open University Press.

Hargreaves, D. (1980). The Occupational Culture of Teachers. In P. Woods (ed.), *Teacher Strategies: explorations in the sociology of the School.* London: Croom Helm.

Harré, R. (1982). Theoretical preliminaries to the study of action. In M. von Cranach & R. Harré (eds.), *The analysis of action: Recent theoretical and empirical advances.* Cambridge, England: Cambridge University Press.

Harrison, R. (1962). Defenses and the Need to Know. *Human Relations Training News,* 6, 4, 266-272.

Henderson, E.S. (1979). The Concept of School-focused In-service Education and Training. *The British Journal of Teacher Education,* 5, 18-25.

Henderson, E.S. and Perry, G.W. (1981). *Change and Development in Schools.* London: McGraw-Hill.

Hewton, E. (1988). *School Focused Staff Development.* Lewes: Falmer Press.

Hopkins, D. (ed.). *In-Service Training and Educational Development: an international survey.* Beckenham: Croom, Helm.

House, E.R. (1981). Three perspectives on innovation. In R. Lehming and M. Kane (eds.), *Improving Schools: Using What we Know.* London: Sage.

Hoyle, E. (1970). Planned organisational change in education. *Research in Education,* 3, May, 1-22.

Hoyle, E. (1973). Strategies of Curriculum Change. In R. Watkins (ed.), *In-Service Training: Structure and Change.* London: Ward Lock.

Hughes, E.C. (1971). Professions. In E.C. Hughes (ed.), *The sociological eye: selected papers.* Chicago: Aldine-Ashton.

Hustler, D., Cassidy, A., and Cuff, E.C. (eds.) (1984). *Action Research in Classrooms and Schools.* London: Allen & Unwin.

Jackson, P. (1968). *Life in Classrooms.* New York: Holt, Rinehart & Winston.

Kemmis, S. (1981). *The Professional Development of Teachers through Involvement in Action-Research Projects.* Geelong, Australia: Deakin University Press.

Kemmis, S. and McTaggart, R. (1981). *The Action Research Planner.* Geelong, Australia: Deakin University Press.

King, R. (1978). *All Things Bright and Beautiful: a sociological study of infant schools.* Chichester: Wiley.

Kristeva, Julia. (1985). The Speaking Subject. In Marshall Blonsky (ed.), *On Signs.* Oxford: Basil Blackwell.

Kroath, F. (1989). How do teachers change their practical theories? *Cambridge Journal of Education,* 19:1, 59-70.

Laat, W.A.M. de. (1985). Vragen naar de onbekende weg. In H. Letiche (Ed.), *From Europe to the teaching team.* Delft, The Netherlands: Eburon.

Laycock, P. (1988). *Branston Trist: Learning about Learning* [Report March]. Lincolnshire, England: Branston School.

Lentz, Leo. (1988). Zelf-evaluatie en het schoolwerkplan. In H. Letiche (Ed.), *Zelf Evaluatie. Een instrument voor onderwijsgevenden en trainers.* Assen: van Gorcum.

Letiche, H. (Ed.) (1985). *From Europe to the Teaching Team.* Delft: EBURON.

Letiche, H. (1988a). Interactive Experiential Learning in Enquiry Courses. In Jennifer Nias (ed.), *The Enquiring Teacher: Supporting and Sustaining Teacher Research.* Sussex: Falmer Press.

Letiche, H. (ed.) (1988b). *Zelf-Evaluatie*. Assen: van Gorcum.

Lieberman, A. (ed.) (1988). *Building a Professional Culture in Schools*. New York: Teachers' College Press.

Lincoln, Y.S. & Guba, E.G. (1985). *Naturalistic inquiry*. Beverley Hills: Sage.

Lortie, D. (1969). The balance of Control and Autonomy in Elementary School Teaching. In A. Etzioni (ed.), *The Semi-Professions and Their Organization*. New York: Free press.

Lortie, D. (1975). *School Teacher: A sociological study*. Chicago: University of Chicago Press.

Lövlie, L. (1974). Pedagogisk filosofi for praktiserende lerere. *Pedagogen*, 1, 19-36.

Lynch, M. (1985). *Art and artefact in labor science: A study of shop work and shop talk*. London: Routledge & Kegan Paul.

Mark Hanson, E. (1985). *Educational administration and organizational behavior*. Boston: Allyn and Baron.

McClelland, D. (1976). *A Guide to Job-Competency Assessment*. Boston: McBeer & Co.

Miles, H. (1983). Unravelling the Mystery of Institutionalisation. *Eductional Leadership*. November.

Miles, M.B. & Huberman, A.M. (1984). *Qualitative data analysis: a source book of new methods*. Beverley Hills: Sage.

Ministerie van Onderwijs en Wetenschappen (1988). Conceptbeleidsnotitie: *Nascholing in het primair en het voortgezet onderwijs*. Den Haag: Staatsuitgeverij.

Ministerie van Onderwijs en Wetenschappen (1989). *Nascholing in het primair en het voortgezet onderwijs*. Den Haag: Staatsuitgeverij.

Ministerie van Onderwijs en Wetenschappen (1990). *Review van het onderwijsbeleid in Nederland: Verslagen en Vragen. OECD rapportage*. Den Haag: Staatsuitgeverij.

Mintzberg, H. (1979). *The structuring of organizations*. Englewood Cliffs: Prentice Hall.

Nias, J. (1987a). Learning from difference: A collegial approach to change. In W.J. Smyth (ed.), *Educating Teachers: Changing the nature of pedagogical knowledge*. London: Falmer Press.

Nias, J. (1987b). *Seeing Anew: Teachers' theories in action*. Geelong: Deakin University Press.

Nias, J. (1989). *Primary Teachers Talking: A study of teaching as work*. London: Routledge.

Nias, J. & Groundwater Smith, S. (eds.) (1988). *The Enquiring Teacher: Sustaining and supporting teacher research*. London: Falmer Press.

Nixon, J. (ed.) (1980). *A Teacher's Guide to Action Research*. London: Grant McIntyre.

Nixon, J. (1987). Only connect: Thoughts on stylistic interchange within the research community. *British Educational Research Journal*, 191-202.

Oja, S.N. and Smulyan, L. (1989). *Collaborative Action Research: A developmental approach*. London: Falmer Press.

Ovens, P., PhD in progress, Manchester Polytechnic.

Peters, R.S. (1966). *Ethics and Education*. London: Allen & Unwin.

Plooij, F.X., & Dungen, M.G.M. van den. (eds.) (1985). *Hulpverleningspraktijk en dienstverlenend onderzoek*. Lisse: Swets & Zeitlinger.

Polanyi, M. (1958). *Personal Knowledge*. London: Routledge & Kegan Paul.

Polanyi, M. (1967). *The tacit dimension*. London: Routledge & Kegan Paul.

Pollard, A. (1985). *The Social World of the Primary School*. London: Cassell.

Rapaport, P. (1970). Three dilemmas in action research. *Human Relations*, 23.

Ribbins, P. (1986). Qualitative Perspectives in Research in Secondary Education. In T. Simpkins (ed.), *Research in the Management of Education*. Sheffield City Polytechnic Papers in Educational Management.

Rudduck, J. & Hopkins, D. (1985). *Research as a Basis for Teaching: Readings from the work of Lawrence Stenhouse*. London: Heinemann Educational Books.

Ryle, G. (1949). *The concept of mind*. London: Hutchinson's University Library.

Sacks, Harvey. (1977). On doing 'Being ordinary'. In J. Maxwell Atkinson & John Heritage (eds.), *Structures of Social Action* Cambridge: Cambridge University Press.

Schein, E. (1983). *Organisasjonskultur og ledelse. Er kulturendring mulig*. Oslo: Mercury Media.

Schmuck, R.A. and Schmuck, P.A. (1974). *A Humanistic Psychology of Eduction*. Mayfield: National Press Books.

Schon, D. (1983). *The Reflective Practitioner*. London: Temple Smith.

Schon, D. (1983). *The Reflective Practitioner: How Professionals Think in Action*. New York: Basic Books.

Schon, D. (1987). *Educating the Reflective Practitioner*. London: Jossey-Bass.

Showers, B., Joyce, B. & Bennett, B. (1987). Synthesis of Research on Staff Development: A Framework for Future Study and a State-of-the-Art Analysis. *Educational Leadership*, 40, (3), 77-87.

Shumsky, A. (1958). The personal significance of action research. *Journal of Teacher Education*. 9, 152-155.

Simons, H. (1979). Suggestions for a school self-evaluation based on democratic principles. In J. Elliott (ed.), *School-based evaluation [specialissue]. Classroom Action Research Network Bulletin*. No. 3. Cambridge Institute of Education.

Smyth, J. (1987). *A Rationale for Teachers' Critical Pedagogy: A Handbook*. Geelong, Australia: Deakin University Press.

Smyth, W.J. (1984). Teachers as collaborative learners. Clinical Supervision: A state of the art review. *Journal of Education for Teaching*, 10 (1).

Steele, F. (1975). *Consulting for Organisation Change*. Amherst, MA: Massachusetts Press.

Stenhouse, L. (1971). Humanities Curriculum Project: The rationale. *Theory into Practice*, 10, 154-162.

Stenhouse, L. (1975). *An Introduction to Curriculum Research and Development*. London: Heinemann.

Stuyts, M. & Grubben, L. (1990). Het onderzoek 'Leren Hulpverlenen': Een ontmoeting tussen opleiding-werkveld-onderzoek. *K & O Tijdschrift*, 33 (5), 20-25.

Taylor, W. (1975). The Universities and In-Service Education. *British Journal of In-Service Education and Training*, 1, 5-6.

Thompson, A. (1984). The use of video as an observation tool. In L. Thompson and A. Thompson (eds.), *What Learning Looks Like: Helping individual teachers to become more effective*. Schools Council Programme 2. London: Longmans.

Tickle, L. (1987). *Learning Teaching, Teaching, Teaching ... A Study of Partnership in Teacher Education*. Lewes: The Falmer Press.

Tulder, M. van, Veenman, S. & Roelofs, E. (1989). *Nascholing leraren basisonderwijs: Vormgeving en resultaten*. Den Haag: SVO.

Wallace, M. (1987). A Historial Review of Action Research: Some implications for the education of teachers in their managerial role. *Journal of Education for Teaching*, 13 (2).

Waller, W. (1961). (new edn.) *Sociology of Teaching*. New York: Russell & Russell.

Watson, L. (1976). A Caring Community: Staff Development in the School. *Secondary Education*, 6, 18-20.

Weick, Karl. (1979). *The Social Psychology of Organizing,* 2nd edition. New York: Random House.

Weick, Karl E. (1982). Administering education in loosely coupled schools. *Phi Delta Kappan*, 64, 673-676.

Wieringen, A.M.L. van. (1989). *Bestuur en Management van Onderwijsinstellingen*. Groningen: Wolters-Noordhoff.

Williams, F. (1987). *Curriculum Descriptions* [Mimeo]. Lincolnshire: Branston School.

Woods, P. (1979). *The Divided School*. London: Routledge & Kegan Paul.

Woods, P. (ed.) (1989). *Working for Teacher Development*. Ely: Peter Francis.

Ziman, J. (1984). *An introduction to science: The philosophical and social aspects of science and technology*. Cambridge: Cambridge University Press.

Ziman, J. (1988). Science in a Steady State. *The Guardian*. 5 April, p 4.